The Complete Anti-Inflammatory Vegan Cookbook

Reduce Inflammation, Optimize Your Gut Health, Fortify Your Immune System, and Detoxify Your Body with Delicious Plant-Based Recipes

Amanda K. Sanders

Table of Contents

Introduction

Say Hello to the Anti-Inflammatory Lifestyle

Welcome aboard an exciting and delicious plant-based anti-inflammatory journey with this cookbook, *"The Complete Anti-Inflammatory Vegan Cookbook"* by Amanda K. Sanders. If you're new to the world of anti-inflammatory eating or looking to expand your culinary repertoire, this book is your ultimate guide to embracing a lifestyle that fights off chronic inflammation and nourishes your body while delighting your taste buds as well. An anti-inflammatory diet can have several benefits, including alleviating chronic pain, boosting the immune system, and promoting overall wellness.

The journey to a vegan-centric anti-inflammatory lifestyle goes beyond simply avoiding specific foods. It also involves embracing a nourishing, plant-based diet that is nutrient-rich to enhance your body's natural defense mechanisms. By adopting a vegan lifestyle, you are embracing a compassionate and environmentally conscious way of eating. This cookbook strives to ensure a smooth and delightful transition, offering delicious recipes that demonstrate how healthy eating can be both gratifying and flavorful.

How to Use This Cookbook

This cookbook is structured to walk you step-by-step through the fundamentals of an anti-inflammatory vegan diet, providing practical advice and several delectable vegan-centric, inflammation-fighting recipes to choose from. Here's how to make the most of it:

1. **Understanding the Basics:** Start with the chapter "Understanding the Anti-Inflammatory Vegan Diet" to grasp the fundamental concepts. Learn what inflammation is, how it affects your health, and why a vegan diet can be particularly effective in combating it.

2. **Sustainable Lifestyle Tips:** Before diving into the recipes, read "Tips for a Sustainable Anti-Inflammatory Vegan Lifestyle." This section provides essential strategies for meal planning, shopping, and staying motivated, ensuring your new lifestyle is both manageable and enjoyable.

3. **Diverse Recipes:** The cookbook is divided into sections based on meal types, from breakfast to desserts. Each recipe is crafted to include anti-inflammatory ingredients, providing you with various options to keep your meals exciting and nutritious.

4. **Meal Plans:** To help you get started, we've included a 30-day meal plan. This resource is designed to take the guesswork out of meal preparation, making it easier to stick to your new eating habits.

5. **Nutritional Information:** Each recipe includes detailed nutritional information, helping you track your intake and ensure you're meeting your dietary needs.

6. **Frequently Asked Questions:** The FAQ section addresses common concerns and challenges you might face. It's a handy resource for troubleshooting and finding quick solutions to any issues that arise.

Embarking on an anti-inflammatory vegan lifestyle is a significant step towards better health and well-being. This cookbook supports you every step of the way, offering inspiration, knowledge, and a sense of community. Let's embark on this adventure and celebrate the joy of eating healthily and living vibrantly.

Chapter 1: Understanding the Anti-Inflammatory Vegan Diet

What is Inflammation?

Inflammation is the body's natural response to injury, infection, or harmful stimuli. It is a vital component of the immune system's defensive process, aiding the body's healing and protection. On the other hand, chronic inflammation can result in a variety of health issues. Numerous illnesses, including diabetes, heart disease, arthritis, and even some types of cancer, have been related to chronic inflammation.

Fundamentally, inflammation is characterized by redness, swelling, heat, and discomfort in the affected area. The immune system triggers this response by releasing chemicals like cytokines and prostaglandins that aid in isolating and eliminating harmful agents. Acute inflammation aids the body in the short term by reacting to harmful foreign agents entering the body and attempting to destroy them, whereas chronic inflammation results from a prolonged inflammatory response, which can damage healthy body cells.

Benefits of an Anti-Inflammatory Diet

The goal of an anti-inflammatory diet is to eat foods that support general health and help lower inflammation. Listed below are some of the main benefits of this diet:

1. **Reduced Risk of Chronic Diseases:** By minimizing inflammation, this diet can lower the risk of chronic diseases such as heart disease, diabetes, and cancer. It can also help manage conditions like arthritis and inflammatory bowel disease.

2. **Improved Digestive Health:** Anti-inflammatory foods support a balanced gut microbiota, enhancing nutrition absorption and digestion. This can help with the symptoms of other digestive illnesses, such as irritable bowel syndrome (IBS).

3. **Enhanced Immune Function:** A diet rich in anti-inflammatory foods helps fortify the immune system, increasing its capacity to fight infections and diseases.

4. **Improved Weight Management:** Several anti-inflammatory foods are nutrient-dense and low-calorie, helping to control weight and lower the risk of obesity-related illnesses.

5. **Improved Energy Levels:** This diet can increase energy and general vitality by lowering inflammation and enhancing nutrient absorption.

Why Choose a Vegan Anti-Inflammatory Diet?

A vegan-based anti-inflammatory diet offers a comprehensive approach to health and wellness by fusing the principles of plant-based nutrition and anti-inflammatory foods. Here's why it's a powerful choice:

1. **Rich in Nutrients:** Diets high in vitamins, minerals, antioxidants, and fiber are commonly associated with veganism. These nutrients are essential for lowering inflammation and promoting general health.

2. **Lower in Saturated Fats:** Plant-based diets are lower in saturated fats, which are primarily found in animal-related foods and can trigger inflammation.

3. **Ethical and Sustainable:** Adopting a vegan diet is also a compassionate choice that promotes environmental sustainability and animal welfare. It encourages a more moral way of living and reduces the carbon footprint.

4. **Better Digestion:** Plant-based foods are often easier to digest and can help with gut health, which is closely linked to inflammation.

5. **Diverse and Flavorful:** A vegan-based anti-inflammatory diet encourages the consumption of a wide variety of fruits, vegetables, whole grains, nuts, seeds, and legumes, which results in a diversified and delightful diet.

Foods to Embrace and Avoid

Foods to Embrace

1. **Fruits and Vegetables:** A diet high in antioxidants and phytonutrients must include fruits and vegetables. Berries, leafy greens, tomatoes, and cruciferous vegetables like broccoli and cauliflower are particularly beneficial.

2. **Whole Grains:** High in fiber and vital nutrients, whole grains like quinoa, brown rice, oats, and barley promote gut health and lower inflammation.

3. **Nuts and Seeds:** Walnuts, almonds, chia seeds, and flaxseeds are great sources of fiber, healthy fats, and anti-inflammatory compounds.

4. **Legumes:** Rich in antioxidants, fiber, and protein, beans, lentils, and chickpeas are a great addition to an anti-inflammatory vegan diet.

5. **Healthy Fats:** Avocados, olive oil, and coconut oil are rich sources of healthy fats that can help reduce inflammation.

6. **Herbs and Spices:** Turmeric, ginger, garlic, and cinnamon, known for their strong anti-inflammatory qualities, can improve the flavor of your dishes.

Foods to Avoid

1. **Processed Foods:** Foods high in artificial additives, refined sugars, and trans fats can exacerbate inflammation. Staying away from fast food, processed snacks, and sugary beverages is critical.

2. **Refined Grains:** Refined grain products, such as white bread and pasta, can worsen inflammation because they lack the fiber and nutrients found in whole grains.

3. **Sugary Foods and Beverages:** Consuming much sugar can trigger inflammatory responses. Limit your soda, candies/sweets, and other sugary treats.

4. **Excessive Alcohol Intake:** While moderate alcohol consumption may have some health benefits, excessive consumption can lead to inflammation and adversely affect overall health.

5. **Certain Vegetable Oils:** Oils high in omega-6 fatty acids, such as corn oil, sunflower oil, and soybean oil, can exacerbate inflammation when used in excess. Choose oils with a better omega-3 to omega-6 ratio, like olive and flaxseed oils.

By prioritizing whole, plant-based meals and avoiding inflammatory triggers, you can create a diet that supports your body's natural defenses and fosters long-term health. This all-encompassing strategy improves general well-being and reduces inflammation, making maintaining a vibrant, healthy lifestyle easier.

Chapter 2: 60-Day Meal Plan

Meal Plan for Days 1-30

Day	Breakfast	Lunch	Dinner	Snack
1	Pineapple Turmeric Smoothie	Quinoa and Avocado Anti-Inflammatory Salad	Eggplant and Chickpea Turmeric Curry	Turmeric Roasted Chickpeas
2	Berry Anti-Inflammatory Blast	Cucumber Mint Detox Salad	Lentil and Vegetable Stir-Fry	Avocado Cilantro Lime Salsa
3	Mango Ginger Green Tea Infusion	Roasted Beet and Walnut Arugula Salad	Spaghetti Squash with Roasted Tomato Sauce	Spiced Edamame Bites
4	Golden Milk Smoothie	Turmeric Tahini Kale Salad	Quinoa-Stuffed Portobello Mushrooms	Sweet Potato and Turmeric Hummus
5	Cucumber Mint Cooler	Blueberry Almond Spinach Salad	Coconut Turmeric Tofu Skewers	Kale Chips with Paprika
6	Blueberry Basil Detox Elixir	Mango Basil Summer Salad	Zucchini Noodles with Creamy Avocado Pesto	Roasted Red Pepper and Walnut Dip
7	Kiwi Turmeric Immunity Smoothie	Roasted Brussels Sprouts and Pomegranate Salad	Sesame Crusted Tofu with Turmeric Citrus Glaze	Sweet Potato and Turmeric Croquettes
8	Green Apple Ginger Detox Elixir	Asparagus and Almond Quinoa Salad	Portobello Mushroom and Spinach Stuffed Peppers	Turmeric Spiced Pumpkin Seeds
9	Anti-Inflammatory Berry Beet Smoothie	Turmeric Mango Cilantro Slaw	Harissa Spiced Chickpea Tagine	Cauliflower Buffalo Bites with Cashew Ranch
10	Pineapple Mint Coconut Water Refresher	Mediterranean Lentil and Artichoke Salad	Coconut Quinoa Pilaf with Roasted Vegetables	Edamame and Mint Guacamole
11	Mango Turmeric Chia Seed Pudding Smoothie	Watermelon Basil Arugula Salad	Lentil Walnut Burger with Avocado Aioli	Sun-Dried Tomato and Basil Hummus
12	Spirulina Citrus Superfood Smoothie	Orange Fennel Detox Salad	Moroccan Spiced Eggplant and Couscous Skillet	Crispy Turmeric Baked Kale Chips
13	Raspberry Turmeric Ginger Smoothie	Avocado Tomato Basil Detox Salad	Walnut and Herb Crusted Tempeh Steaks	Turmeric Hemp Seed Energy Bites
14	Detox Green Tea Infusion with Lemon and Mint	Roasted Cauliflower and Cumin Chickpea Salad	Creamy Turmeric Polenta with Roasted Vegetables	Crispy Baked Turmeric Artichoke Hearts

15	Papaya Turmeric Immunity Elixir	Arugula Pomegranate Quinoa Salad	Moroccan Spiced Lentil and Eggplant Casserole	Miso Glazed Edamame Pods
16	Blueberry Lavender Almond Milk Smoothie	Turmeric Roasted Carrot and Chickpea Salad	Smoky Turmeric Grilled Portobello Mushrooms	Spicy Turmeric Popcorn
17	Pineapple Basil Anti-Inflammatory Cooler	Mango Avocado Black Bean Salad	Spaghetti Squash with Spinach and Pine Nut Pesto	Almond and Turmeric Stuffed Grape Leaves
18	Orange Turmeric Mango Smoothie Bowl	Spinach Strawberry Walnut Salad with Balsamic Vinaigrette	Quinoa and Black Bean Stuffed Bell Peppers	Mediterranean Roasted Red Pepper and Walnut Dip
19	Pineapple Turmeric Smoothie	Quinoa and Avocado Anti-Inflammatory Salad	Eggplant and Chickpea Turmeric Curry	Turmeric Roasted Chickpeas
20	Berry Anti-Inflammatory Blast	Cucumber Mint Detox Salad	Lentil and Vegetable Stir-Fry	Avocado Cilantro Lime Salsa
21	Mango Ginger Green Tea Infusion	Roasted Beet and Walnut Arugula Salad	Spaghetti Squash with Roasted Tomato Sauce	Spiced Edamame Bites
22	Golden Milk Smoothie	Turmeric Tahini Kale Salad	Quinoa-Stuffed Portobello Mushrooms	Sweet Potato and Turmeric Hummus
23	Cucumber Mint Cooler	Blueberry Almond Spinach Salad	Coconut Turmeric Tofu Skewers	Kale Chips with Paprika
24	Blueberry Basil Detox Elixir	Mango Basil Summer Salad	Zucchini Noodles with Creamy Avocado Pesto	Roasted Red Pepper and Walnut Dip
25	Kiwi Turmeric Immunity Smoothie	Roasted Brussels Sprouts and Pomegranate Salad	Sesame Crusted Tofu with Turmeric Citrus Glaze	Sweet Potato and Turmeric Croquettes
26	Green Apple Ginger Detox Elixir	Asparagus and Almond Quinoa Salad	Portobello Mushroom and Spinach Stuffed Peppers	Turmeric Spiced Pumpkin Seeds
27	Anti-Inflammatory Berry Beet Smoothie	Turmeric Mango Cilantro Slaw	Harissa Spiced Chickpea Tagine	Cauliflower Buffalo Bites with Cashew Ranch
28	Pineapple Mint Coconut Water Refresher	Mediterranean Lentil and Artichoke Salad	Coconut Quinoa Pilaf with Roasted Vegetables	Edamame and Mint Guacamole
29	Mango Turmeric Chia Seed Pudding Smoothie	Watermelon Basil Arugula Salad	Lentil Walnut Burger with Avocado Aioli	Sun-Dried Tomato and Basil Hummus
30	Spirulina Citrus Superfood Smoothie	Orange Fennel Detox Salad	Moroccan Spiced Eggplant and Couscous Skillet	Crispy Turmeric Baked Kale Chips

Meal Plan for Days 31-60

Day	Breakfast	Lunch	Dinner	Snack
1	Raspberry Turmeric Ginger Smoothie	Avocado Tomato Basil Detox Salad	Walnut and Herb Crusted Tempeh Steaks	Turmeric Hemp Seed Energy Bites
2	Detox Green Tea Infusion with Lemon and Mint	Roasted Cauliflower and Cumin Chickpea Salad	Creamy Turmeric Polenta with Roasted Vegetables	Crispy Baked Turmeric Artichoke Hearts
3	Papaya Turmeric Immunity Elixir	Arugula Pomegranate Quinoa Salad	Moroccan Spiced Lentil and Eggplant Casserole	Miso Glazed Edamame Pods
4	Blueberry Lavender Almond Milk Smoothie	Turmeric Roasted Carrot and Chickpea Salad	Smoky Turmeric Grilled Portobello Mushrooms	Spicy Turmeric Popcorn
5	Pineapple Basil Anti-Inflammatory Cooler	Mango Avocado Black Bean Salad	Spaghetti Squash with Spinach and Pine Nut Pesto	Almond and Turmeric Stuffed Grape Leaves
6	Orange Turmeric Mango Smoothie Bowl	Spinach Strawberry Walnut Salad with Balsamic Vinaigrette	Quinoa and Black Bean Stuffed Bell Peppers	Mediterranean Roasted Red Pepper and Walnut Dip
7	Pineapple Turmeric Smoothie	Quinoa and Avocado Anti-Inflammatory Salad	Eggplant and Chickpea Turmeric Curry	Turmeric Roasted Chickpeas
8	Berry Anti-Inflammatory Blast	Cucumber Mint Detox Salad	Lentil and Vegetable Stir-Fry	Avocado Cilantro Lime Salsa
9	Mango Ginger Green Tea Infusion	Roasted Beet and Walnut Arugula Salad	Spaghetti Squash with Roasted Tomato Sauce	Spiced Edamame Bites
10	Golden Milk Smoothie	Turmeric Tahini Kale Salad	Quinoa-Stuffed Portobello Mushrooms	Sweet Potato and Turmeric Hummus
11	Cucumber Mint Cooler	Blueberry Almond Spinach Salad	Coconut Turmeric Tofu Skewers	Kale Chips with Paprika

12	Blueberry Basil Detox Elixir	Mango Basil Summer Salad	Zucchini Noodles with Creamy Avocado Pesto	Roasted Red Pepper and Walnut Dip
13	Kiwi Turmeric Immunity Smoothie	Roasted Brussels Sprouts and Pomegranate Salad	Sesame Crusted Tofu with Turmeric Citrus Glaze	Sweet Potato and Turmeric Croquettes
14	Green Apple Ginger Detox Elixir	Asparagus and Almond Quinoa Salad	Portobello Mushroom and Spinach Stuffed Peppers	Turmeric Spiced Pumpkin Seeds
15	Anti-Inflammatory Berry Beet Smoothie	Turmeric Mango Cilantro Slaw	Harissa Spiced Chickpea Tagine	Cauliflower Buffalo Bites with Cashew Ranch
16	Pineapple Mint Coconut Water Refresher	Mediterranean Lentil and Artichoke Salad	Coconut Quinoa Pilaf with Roasted Vegetables	Edamame and Mint Guacamole
17	Mango Turmeric Chia Seed Pudding Smoothie	Watermelon Basil Arugula Salad	Lentil Walnut Burger with Avocado Aioli	Sun-Dried Tomato and Basil Hummus
18	Spirulina Citrus Superfood Smoothie	Orange Fennel Detox Salad	Moroccan Spiced Eggplant and Couscous Skillet	Crispy Turmeric Baked Kale Chips
19	Raspberry Turmeric Ginger Smoothie	Avocado Tomato Basil Detox Salad	Walnut and Herb Crusted Tempeh Steaks	Turmeric Hemp Seed Energy Bites
20	Detox Green Tea Infusion with Lemon and Mint	Roasted Cauliflower and Cumin Chickpea Salad	Creamy Turmeric Polenta with Roasted Vegetables	Crispy Baked Turmeric Artichoke Hearts
21	Papaya Turmeric Immunity Elixir	Arugula Pomegranate Quinoa Salad	Moroccan Spiced Lentil and Eggplant Casserole	Miso Glazed Edamame Pods
22	Blueberry Lavender Almond Milk Smoothie	Turmeric Roasted Carrot and Chickpea Salad	Smoky Turmeric Grilled Portobello Mushrooms	Spicy Turmeric Popcorn

23	Pineapple Basil Anti-Inflammatory Cooler	Mango Avocado Black Bean Salad	Spaghetti Squash with Spinach and Pine Nut Pesto	Almond and Turmeric Stuffed Grape Leaves
24	Orange Turmeric Mango Smoothie Bowl	Spinach Strawberry Walnut Salad with Balsamic Vinaigrette	Quinoa and Black Bean Stuffed Bell Peppers	Mediterranean Roasted Red Pepper and Walnut Dip
25	Pineapple Turmeric Smoothie	Quinoa and Avocado Anti-Inflammatory Salad	Eggplant and Chickpea Turmeric Curry	Turmeric Roasted Chickpeas
26	Berry Anti-Inflammatory Blast	Cucumber Mint Detox Salad	Lentil and Vegetable Stir-Fry	Avocado Cilantro Lime Salsa
27	Mango Ginger Green Tea Infusion	Roasted Beet and Walnut Arugula Salad	Spaghetti Squash with Roasted Tomato Sauce	Spiced Edamame Bites
28	Golden Milk Smoothie	Turmeric Tahini Kale Salad	Quinoa-Stuffed Portobello Mushrooms	Sweet Potato and Turmeric Hummus
29	Cucumber Mint Cooler	Blueberry Almond Spinach Salad	Coconut Turmeric Tofu Skewers	Kale Chips with Paprika
30	Blueberry Basil Detox Elixir	Mango Basil Summer Salad	Zucchini Noodles with Creamy Avocado Pesto	Roasted Red Pepper and Walnut Dip

Chapter 3: Soups and Stews

Turmeric Lentil Soup

Prep Time: 15 minutes | **Cook Time:** 40 minutes | **Servings:** 4

Ingredients:

- 1 cup dried green lentils
- 1 large onion, finely chopped
- 2 carrots, peeled and diced
- 2 celery stalks, sliced
- 3 cloves garlic, minced
- 1 tablespoon grated fresh ginger
- 1 teaspoon ground turmeric
- 1 teaspoon ground cumin
- 1 teaspoon ground coriander
- 1/2 teaspoon ground cinnamon
- 4 cups vegetable broth
- 1 can (14 ounces) diced tomatoes
- 1 cup kale, stems removed and leaves chopped
- Salt and pepper to taste
- 2 tablespoons olive oil
- Fresh cilantro for garnish

Instructions:

1. Rinse the green lentils under cold water and set aside.

2. In a large pot, heat olive oil over medium heat. Add the chopped onion, diced carrots, and sliced celery. Sauté until the vegetables are softened, about 5 minutes.

3. Stir in the minced garlic, grated ginger, ground turmeric, ground cumin, ground coriander, and ground cinnamon. Cook for an additional 2 minutes until the spices become fragrant.

4. Add the rinsed lentils, vegetable broth, and diced tomatoes (with their juice) to the pot. Bring the mixture to a boil, then reduce the heat to low, cover, and simmer for 30 minutes.

5. After simmering, add the chopped kale to the soup. Cook for an additional 5-7 minutes until the kale is tender.

6. Season the soup with salt and pepper to taste. Ladle the soup into bowls and garnish with fresh cilantro.

Nutritional Information (per serving):

- **Carbs:** 35g
- **Fats:** 7g
- **Fiber:** 12g
- **Protein:** 15g

<u>Sweet Potato Ginger Stew</u>

Prep Time: 20 minutes | **Cook Time:** 30 minutes | **Servings:** 6

Ingredients:

- 2 large sweet potatoes, peeled and cubed
- 1 cup dried red lentils
- 1 large onion, finely chopped
- 3 cloves garlic, minced
- 1 tablespoon grated fresh ginger
- 1 teaspoon ground turmeric
- 1 teaspoon ground cumin
- 1/2 teaspoon ground cinnamon
- 4 cups vegetable broth
- 1 can (14 ounces) coconut milk
- 2 tablespoons olive oil
- Salt and pepper to taste
- Fresh cilantro for garnish

Instructions:

1. Peel and cube the sweet potatoes. Set aside.

2. Rinse the red lentils under cold water and set aside.

3. In a large pot, heat olive oil over medium heat. Add the chopped onion and sauté until translucent. Add minced garlic, grated ginger, ground turmeric, ground cumin, and ground cinnamon. Cook for 2-3 minutes until fragrant.

4. Stir in the cubed sweet potatoes and rinsed red lentils. Ensure they are well-coated with the aromatic mixture.

5. Add vegetable broth and coconut milk to the pot. Bring the mixture to a boil, then reduce the heat to low, cover, and simmer for 25-30 minutes or until sweet potatoes and lentils are tender.

6. Season the stew with salt and pepper to taste. Ladle the stew into bowls and garnish with fresh cilantro.

Nutritional Information (per serving):

- **Carbs:** 45g
- **Fats:** 12g
- **Fiber:** 10g
- **Protein:** 9g

Spinach and White Bean Detox Soup

Prep Time: 15 minutes | **Cook Time:** 25 minutes | **Servings:** 4

Ingredients:

- 1 tablespoon olive oil
- 1 large onion, finely chopped
- 3 cloves garlic, minced
- 1 large carrot, peeled and sliced
- 2 celery stalks, sliced
- 1 teaspoon ground turmeric
- 1 teaspoon ground cumin
- 1/2 teaspoon ground coriander
- 4 cups vegetable broth
- 1 can (15 ounces) white beans, drained and rinsed
- 4 cups fresh spinach, stems removed
- 1 cup cherry tomatoes, halved
- Salt and pepper to taste
- Fresh lemon juice for serving
- Fresh parsley for garnish

Instructions:

1. In a large pot, heat olive oil over medium heat. Add the chopped onion, minced garlic, sliced carrot, and sliced celery. Sauté until the vegetables are softened, about 5 minutes.

2. Stir in ground turmeric, ground cumin, and ground coriander. Cook for an additional 2 minutes until the spices become fragrant.

3. Add vegetable broth and drained white beans to the pot. Bring the mixture to a simmer and cook for 15 minutes.

4. Stir in the fresh spinach and halved cherry tomatoes. Cook for an additional 5 minutes until the spinach wilts and the tomatoes soften.

5. Season the soup with salt and pepper to taste. Squeeze fresh lemon juice over each serving and garnish with fresh parsley.

Nutritional Information (per serving):

- **Carbs:** 30g
- **Fats:** 5g
- **Fiber:** 10g
- **Protein:** 8g

Creamy Broccoli Turmeric Soup

Prep Time: 15 minutes | **Cook Time:** 30 minutes | **Servings:** 6

Ingredients:

- 1 tablespoon olive oil
- 1 large onion, finely chopped
- 3 cloves garlic, minced
- 1 head broccoli, florets separated and stems chopped
- 1 large potato, peeled and diced
- 1 teaspoon ground turmeric
- 4 cups vegetable broth
- 1 can (14 ounces) coconut milk
- Salt and pepper to taste
- Fresh chives for garnish

Instructions:

1. In a large pot, heat olive oil over medium heat. Add the chopped onion and minced garlic. Sauté until the onion is translucent.

2. Add the chopped broccoli stems and diced potato to the pot. Stir and cook for 5 minutes.

3. Sprinkle ground turmeric over the vegetables and stir adequately to coat.

4. Add vegetable broth to the pot. Bring the mixture to a boil, then reduce the heat to low, cover, and simmer for 15-20 minutes, or until the vegetables are tender.

5. Use an immersion blender to puree the soup until smooth. Alternatively, transfer the soup in batches to a blender and blend until smooth. Be cautious when blending hot liquids.

6. Stir in the coconut milk and season the soup with salt and pepper to taste. Heat through, but do not boil.

7. Ladle the creamy soup into bowls and garnish with fresh chives.

Nutritional Information (per serving):

- **Carbs:** 25g
- **Fats:** 12g
- **Fiber:** 5g
- **Protein:** 4g

Chickpea and Kale Miso Stew

Prep Time: 15 minutes | **Cook Time:** 25 minutes | **Servings:** 4

Ingredients:

- 1 tablespoon olive oil
- 1 large onion, finely chopped
- 3 cloves garlic, minced
- 1 can (15 ounces) chickpeas, drained and rinsed
- 4 cups vegetable broth
- 1 large sweet potato, peeled and diced
- 1 bunch kale, stems removed and leaves chopped
- 2 tablespoons white miso paste
- 1 teaspoon ground turmeric
- Salt and pepper to taste
- Fresh parsley for garnish

Instructions:

1. In a large pot, heat olive oil over medium heat. Add the chopped onion and minced garlic. Sauté until the onion is translucent.
2. Stir in the drained chickpeas and vegetable broth. Bring the mixture to a boil.
3. Add the diced sweet potato to the pot. Simmer for 15-20 minutes, or until the sweet potato is tender.
4. Stir in the chopped kale leaves. Cook for an additional 5 minutes until the kale is wilted.
5. In a small bowl, dissolve white miso paste in a ladle of hot broth from the stew. Mix adequately to ensure the miso is fully dissolved.
6. Pour the miso mixture back into the pot. Add ground turmeric, salt, and pepper to taste. Stir adequately to combine.
7. Ladle the stew into bowls and garnish with fresh parsley.

Nutritional Information (per serving):

- **Carbs:** 40g
- **Fats:** 8g
- **Fiber:** 10g
- **Protein:** 10g

Butternut Squash Anti-Inflammatory Chowder

Prep Time: 20 minutes | **Cook Time:** 40 minutes | **Servings:** 6

Ingredients:

- 1 tablespoon olive oil
- 1 large onion, finely chopped
- 3 cloves garlic, minced
- 1 butternut squash, peeled, seeded, and diced
- 2 carrots, peeled and sliced
- 2 celery stalks, sliced
- 1 teaspoon ground turmeric
- 1 teaspoon ground ginger
- 4 cups vegetable broth
- 1 can (14 ounces) coconut milk
- Salt and pepper to taste
- Fresh chives for garnish

Instructions:

1. In a large pot, heat olive oil over medium heat. Add the chopped onion and minced garlic. Sauté until the onion is translucent.
2. Stir in the diced butternut squash, sliced carrots, and sliced celery. Cook for 5-7 minutes until the vegetables begin to soften.
3. Sprinkle ground turmeric and ground ginger over the vegetables. Stir adequately to coat.
4. Add vegetable broth and coconut milk to the pot. Bring the mixture to a boil, then reduce the heat to low, cover, and simmer for 30 minutes or until the vegetables are tender.
5. Season the chowder with salt and pepper to taste. Stir adequately.
6. Use an immersion blender to partially blend the chowder, leaving some chunks for texture.
7. Ladle the chowder into bowls and garnish with fresh chives.

Nutritional Information (per serving):

- **Carbs:** 30g
- **Fats:** 12g
- **Fiber:** 7g
- **Protein:** 3g

<u>Red Lentil and Kale Anti-Inflammatory Stew</u>

Prep Time: 15 minutes | **Cook Time:** 30 minutes | **Servings:** 4

Ingredients:

- 1 tablespoon olive oil
- 1 large onion, finely chopped
- 3 cloves garlic, minced
- 1 cup dried red lentils
- 1 large carrot, peeled and diced
- 2 celery stalks, sliced
- 1 teaspoon ground turmeric
- 1 teaspoon ground cumin
- 1/2 teaspoon ground coriander
- 4 cups vegetable broth
- 1 bunch kale, stems removed and leaves chopped
- 1 can (14 ounces) diced tomatoes
- Salt and pepper to taste
- Fresh lemon wedges for serving

Instructions:

1. In a large pot, heat olive oil over medium heat. Add the chopped onion and minced garlic. Sauté until the onion is translucent.

2. Stir in the red lentils, diced carrot, and sliced celery. Cook for 2-3 minutes.

3. Sprinkle ground turmeric, ground cumin, and ground coriander over the vegetables. Stir adequately to combine.

4. Add vegetable broth to the pot. Bring the mixture to a boil, then reduce the heat to low, cover, and simmer for 15-20 minutes or until the lentils are tender.

5. Stir in the chopped kale leaves and diced tomatoes (with their juice). Cook for an additional 5-7 minutes until the kale is wilted.

6. Season the stew with salt and pepper to taste. Stir adequately.

7. Ladle the stew into bowls and serve with fresh lemon wedges on the side.

Nutritional Information (per serving):

- **Carbs:** 45g
- **Fats:** 5g
- **Fiber:** 12g
- **Protein:** 10g

Coconut Curry Cauliflower Soup

Prep Time: 15 minutes | **Cook Time:** 25 minutes | **Servings:** 4

Ingredients:

- 1 tablespoon olive oil
- 1 large onion, finely chopped
- 3 cloves garlic, minced
- 1 head cauliflower, florets separated
- 1 large carrot, peeled and sliced
- 1 teaspoon ground turmeric
- 1 teaspoon curry powder
- 1 can (14 ounces) coconut milk
- 4 cups vegetable broth
- Salt and pepper to taste
- Fresh cilantro for garnish

Instructions:

1. In a large pot, heat olive oil over medium heat. Add the chopped onion and minced garlic. Sauté until the onion is translucent.

2. Stir in the cauliflower florets and sliced carrot. Cook for 5-7 minutes until the vegetables begin to soften.

3. Sprinkle ground turmeric and curry powder over the vegetables. Stir adequately to coat.

4. Add coconut milk and vegetable broth to the pot. Bring the mixture to a boil, then reduce the heat to low, cover, and simmer for 15-20 minutes or until the cauliflower is tender.

5. Season the soup with salt and pepper to taste. Stir adequately.

6. Use an immersion blender to blend the soup until smooth. Alternatively, transfer the soup in batches to a blender and blend until smooth. Be cautious when blending hot liquids.

7. Ladle the soup into bowls and garnish with fresh cilantro.

Nutritional Information (per serving):

- **Carbs:** 20g
- **Fats:** 15g
- **Fiber:** 5g
- **Protein:** 4g

Ginger Lemongrass Butternut Squash Bisque

Prep Time: 20 minutes | **Cook Time:** 40 minutes | **Servings:** 6

Ingredients:

- 1 tablespoon olive oil
- 1 large onion, finely chopped
- 3 cloves garlic, minced
- 1 butternut squash, peeled, seeded, and diced
- 1 large carrot, peeled and sliced
- 1 stalk lemongrass, bruised and sliced
- 1 tablespoon fresh ginger, grated
- 4 cups vegetable broth
- 1 can (14 ounces) coconut milk
- 1 teaspoon ground turmeric
- Salt and pepper to taste
- Fresh cilantro for garnish

Instructions:

1. In a large pot, heat olive oil over medium heat. Add the chopped onion and minced garlic. Sauté until the onion is translucent.

2. Stir in the diced butternut squash and sliced carrot. Cook for 5-7 minutes until the vegetables begin to soften.

3. Add the sliced lemongrass and grated ginger to the pot. Stir adequately to infuse the flavors.

4. Add vegetable broth and coconut milk to the pot. Bring the mixture to a boil, then reduce the heat to low, cover, and simmer for 30 minutes or until the vegetables are tender.

5. Sprinkle ground turmeric over the soup and season with salt and pepper to taste. Stir adequately.

6. Use an immersion blender to blend the bisque until smooth. Alternatively, transfer the bisque in batches to a blender and blend until smooth. Be cautious when blending hot liquids.

7. Ladle the bisque into bowls and garnish with fresh cilantro.

Nutritional Information (per serving):

- **Carbs:** 25g
- **Fats:** 10g
- **Fiber:** 5g
- **Protein:** 3g

Quinoa Vegetable Turmeric Congee

Prep Time: 15 minutes | **Cook Time:** 30 minutes | **Servings:** 4

Ingredients:

- 1 cup quinoa, rinsed
- 6 cups vegetable broth
- 1 carrot, peeled and sliced
- 1 zucchini, diced
- 1 cup spinach, chopped
- 1 teaspoon ground turmeric
- 1 tablespoon fresh ginger, grated
- 1 tablespoon tamari (gluten-free soy sauce)
- Salt and pepper to taste
- Green onions for garnish
- Sesame seeds for garnish

Instructions:

1. Rinse quinoa under cold water and set aside.

2. In a large pot, combine quinoa and vegetable broth. Bring to a boil, then reduce the heat to low, cover, and simmer for 15 minutes.

3. Stir in the sliced carrot, diced zucchini, chopped spinach, ground turmeric, and grated ginger. Cook for an additional 10-15 minutes until the vegetables are tender.

4. Add tamari (gluten-free soy sauce) to the congee. Season with salt and pepper to taste. Stir adequately to combine.

5. Ladle the congee into bowls and garnish with chopped green onions and sesame seeds.

Nutritional Information (per serving):

- **Carbs:** 40g
- **Fats:** 6g
- **Fiber:** 7g
- **Protein:** 10g

<u>Spicy Black Bean and Spinach Detox Soup</u>

Prep Time: 15 minutes | **Cook Time:** 30 minutes | **Servings:** 4

Ingredients:

- 1 tablespoon olive oil
- 1 large onion, finely chopped
- 3 cloves garlic, minced
- 2 cans (15 ounces each) black beans, drained and rinsed
- 1 can (14 ounces) diced tomatoes
- 4 cups vegetable broth
- 1 teaspoon ground cumin
- 1 teaspoon chili powder
- 1/2 teaspoon cayenne pepper
- 4 cups fresh spinach, chopped
- Juice of 1 lime
- Salt and pepper to taste
- Fresh cilantro for garnish
- Avocado slices for topping

Instructions:

1. In a large pot, heat olive oil over medium heat. Add the chopped onion and minced garlic. Sauté until the onion is translucent.

2. Stir in the drained black beans and diced tomatoes (with their juice). Cook for 5-7 minutes.

3. Add vegetable broth to the pot. Bring the mixture to a boil, then reduce the heat to low, cover, and simmer for 15 minutes.

4. Sprinkle ground cumin, chili powder, and cayenne pepper over the soup. Stir adequately to incorporate the spices.

5. Add the chopped spinach and lime juice to the pot. Cook for an additional 5 minutes until the spinach wilts.

6. Season the soup with salt and pepper to taste. Stir adequately.

7. Ladle the soup into bowls and garnish with fresh cilantro. Top with avocado slices.

Nutritional Information (per serving):

- **Carbs:** 35g
- **Fats:** 6g
- **Fiber:** 12g
- **Protein:** 10g

Creamy Turmeric Coconut Carrot Soup

Prep Time: 15 minutes | **Cook Time:** 30 minutes | **Servings:** 4

Ingredients:

- 1 tablespoon coconut oil
- 1 large onion, finely chopped
- 3 cloves garlic, minced
- 1 pound carrots, peeled and sliced
- 1 teaspoon ground turmeric
- 4 cups vegetable broth
- 1 can (14 ounces) coconut milk
- 1 tablespoon fresh ginger, grated
- Salt and pepper to taste
- Fresh cilantro for garnish
- Coconut cream for drizzling

Instructions:

1. In a large pot, heat coconut oil over medium heat. Add the chopped onion and minced garlic. Sauté until the onion is translucent.

2. Stir in the sliced carrots and ground turmeric. Cook for 5-7 minutes until the carrots start to soften.

3. Add vegetable broth and coconut milk to the pot. Bring the mixture to a boil, then reduce the heat to low, cover, and simmer for 20 minutes or until the carrots are tender.

4. Add grated fresh ginger to the soup. Stir adequately to infuse the flavors.

5. Use an immersion blender to blend the soup until smooth. Alternatively, transfer the soup in batches to a blender and blend until smooth. Be cautious when blending hot liquids.

6. Season the soup with salt and pepper to taste. Stir adequately.

7. Ladle the soup into bowls and garnish with fresh cilantro. Drizzle with coconut cream before serving.

Nutritional Information (per serving):

- **Carbs:** 20g
- **Fats:** 15g
- **Fiber:** 5g
- **Protein:** 2g

Lemon Rosemary White Bean Soup

Prep Time: 15 minutes | **Cook Time:** 25 minutes | **Servings:** 4

Ingredients:

- 1 tablespoon olive oil
- 1 large onion, finely chopped
- 3 cloves garlic, minced
- 2 cans (15 ounces each) white beans, drained and rinsed
- 4 cups vegetable broth
- 1 sprig fresh rosemary
- 1 lemon, juiced and zested
- Salt and pepper to taste
- Fresh parsley for garnish

Instructions:

1. In a large pot, heat olive oil over medium heat. Add the chopped onion and minced garlic. Sauté until the onion is translucent.

2. Stir in the drained white beans and vegetable broth. Bring the mixture to a boil, then reduce the heat to low, cover, and simmer for 15 minutes.

3. Add the sprig of fresh rosemary to the pot. Allow it to infuse its flavor into the soup while simmering.

4. Squeeze the juice of one lemon into the soup and add the lemon zest. Stir adequately to incorporate the citrusy flavors.

5. Season the soup with salt and pepper to taste. Take out the rosemary sprig.

6. Ladle the soup into bowls and garnish with fresh parsley.

Nutritional Information (per serving):

- **Carbs:** 35g
- **Fats:** 6g
- **Fiber:** 9g
- **Protein:** 8g

Spiced Pumpkin and Lentil Stew

Prep Time: 20 minutes | **Cook Time:** 40 minutes | **Servings:** 6

Ingredients:

- 1 tablespoon olive oil
- 1 large onion, finely chopped
- 3 cloves garlic, minced
- 1 pumpkin (about 3 pounds), peeled, seeded, and diced
- 1 cup dried green lentils, rinsed
- 1 can (14 ounces) diced tomatoes
- 4 cups vegetable broth
- 1 teaspoon ground turmeric
- 1 teaspoon ground cumin
- 1/2 teaspoon ground cinnamon
- Salt and pepper to taste
- Fresh cilantro for garnish

Instructions:

1. In a large pot, heat olive oil over medium heat. Add the chopped onion and minced garlic. Sauté until the onion is translucent.

2. Stir in the diced pumpkin and rinsed green lentils. Cook for 5-7 minutes until the pumpkin starts to soften.

3. Add diced tomatoes (with their juice) and vegetable broth to the pot. Bring the mixture to a boil, then reduce the heat to low, cover, and simmer for 30 minutes or until the pumpkin and lentils are tender.

4. Sprinkle ground turmeric, ground cumin, and ground cinnamon over the stew. Stir adequately to incorporate the spices.

5. Season the stew with salt and pepper to taste. Stir adequately.

6. Ladle the stew into bowls and garnish with fresh cilantro.

Nutritional Information (per serving):

- **Carbs:** 40g
- **Fats:** 5g
- **Fiber:** 12g
- **Protein:** 10g

Creamy Turmeric Mushroom Bisque

Prep Time: 15 minutes | **Cook Time:** 30 minutes | **Servings:** 4

Ingredients:

- 1 tablespoon olive oil
- 1 large onion, finely chopped
- 3 cloves garlic, minced
- 1 pound mushrooms, sliced
- 1 teaspoon ground turmeric
- 4 cups vegetable broth
- 1 can (14 ounces) coconut milk
- 1 tablespoon nutritional yeast
- Salt and pepper to taste
- Fresh thyme for garnish

Instructions:

1. In a large pot, heat olive oil over medium heat. Add the chopped onion and minced garlic. Sauté until the onion is translucent.

2. Stir in the sliced mushrooms and cook for 5-7 minutes until they release their moisture and start to brown.

3. Sprinkle ground turmeric over the mushrooms. Stir adequately to coat.

4. Add vegetable broth and coconut milk to the pot. Bring the mixture to a boil, then reduce the heat to low, cover, and simmer for 15-20 minutes.

5. Stir in nutritional yeast to add a cheesy flavor to the bisque. Season with salt and pepper to taste. Stir adequately.

6. Use an immersion blender to blend the bisque until smooth. Alternatively, transfer the bisque in batches to a blender and blend until smooth. Be cautious when blending hot liquids.

7. Ladle the bisque into bowls and garnish with fresh thyme.

Nutritional Information (per serving):

- **Carbs:** 12g
- **Fats:** 15g
- **Fiber:** 3g
- **Protein:** 4g

Thai-Inspired Lemongrass Coconut Soup

Prep Time: 20 minutes | **Cook Time:** 30 minutes | **Servings:** 4

Ingredients:

- 1 tablespoon coconut oil
- 1 large onion, finely chopped
- 3 cloves garlic, minced
- 2 lemongrass stalks, bruised and sliced
- 1 red bell pepper, sliced
- 1 carrot, julienned
- 8 ounces shiitake mushrooms, sliced
- 4 cups vegetable broth
- 1 can (14 ounces) coconut milk
- 1 tablespoon tamari (gluten-free soy sauce)
- 1 tablespoon agave syrup
- Juice of 2 limes
- Salt and pepper to taste
- Fresh cilantro for garnish
- Thai basil leaves for garnish
- Red chili slices for garnish (optional)

Instructions:

1. In a large pot, heat coconut oil over medium heat. Add the chopped onion and minced garlic. Sauté until the onion is translucent.

2. Stir in the sliced lemongrass, red bell pepper, and julienned carrot. Cook for 5-7 minutes until the vegetables start to soften.

3. Add the sliced shiitake mushrooms to the pot. Cook for an additional 3-5 minutes.

4. Add vegetable broth and coconut milk to the pot. Bring the mixture to a boil, then reduce the heat to low, cover, and simmer for 15-20 minutes.

5. Stir in tamari, agave syrup, and the juice of 2 limes. Season with salt and pepper to taste. Adjust the flavors to your liking.

6. Ladle the soup into bowls and garnish with fresh cilantro, Thai basil leaves, and red chili slices (if using).

Nutritional Information (per serving):

- **Carbs:** 20g
- **Fats:** 15g
- **Fiber:** 5g
- **Protein:** 3g

Golden Split Pea and Sweet Potato Stew

Prep Time: 15 minutes | **Cook Time:** 40 minutes | **Servings:** 6

Ingredients:

- 1 tablespoon olive oil
- 1 large onion, finely chopped
- 3 cloves garlic, minced
- 1 cup dried split peas, rinsed and drained
- 2 sweet potatoes, peeled and diced
- 1 teaspoon ground turmeric
- 1 teaspoon ground cumin
- 1/2 teaspoon smoked paprika
- 6 cups vegetable broth
- Salt and pepper to taste
- Fresh parsley for garnish
- Lemon wedges for serving

Instructions:

1. In a large pot, heat olive oil over medium heat. Add the chopped onion and minced garlic. Sauté until the onion is translucent.

2. Stir in the dried split peas and diced sweet potatoes. Cook for 5-7 minutes until the sweet potatoes start to soften.

3. Sprinkle ground turmeric, ground cumin, and smoked paprika over the vegetables. Stir adequately to coat.

4. Add vegetable broth to the pot. Bring the mixture to a boil, then reduce the heat to low, cover, and simmer for 30 minutes or until the split peas and sweet potatoes are tender.

5. Season the stew with salt and pepper to taste. Stir adequately.

6. Ladle the stew into bowls and garnish with fresh parsley. Serve with lemon wedges on the side.

Nutritional Information (per serving):

- **Carbs:** 45g
- **Fats:** 3g
- **Fiber:** 12g
- **Protein:** 10g

Quinoa Minestrone with Kale and Cannellini Beans

Prep Time: 20 minutes | **Cook Time:** 35 minutes | **Servings:** 6

Ingredients:

- 1 tablespoon olive oil
- 1 large onion, finely chopped
- 3 cloves garlic, minced
- 2 carrots, peeled and sliced
- 2 celery stalks, sliced
- 1 zucchini, diced
- 1 cup quinoa, rinsed
- 1 can (14 ounces) diced tomatoes
- 6 cups vegetable broth
- 1 teaspoon dried oregano
- 1 teaspoon dried basil
- 1 bay leaf
- 1 can (14 ounces) cannellini beans, drained and rinsed
- 2 cups kale, stems removed and chopped
- Salt and pepper to taste
- Fresh parsley for garnish
- Vegan Parmesan for serving (optional)

Instructions:

1. In a large pot, heat olive oil over medium heat. Add the chopped onion and minced garlic. Sauté until the onion is translucent.

2. Stir in the sliced carrots, celery, and diced zucchini. Cook for 5-7 minutes until the vegetables start to soften.

3. Add the rinsed quinoa and diced tomatoes (with their juice) to the pot. Stir adequately.

4. Add vegetable broth, dried oregano, dried basil, and the bay leaf to the pot. Bring the mixture to a boil, then reduce the heat to low, cover, and simmer for 15 minutes.

5. Stir in the drained and rinsed cannellini beans and chopped kale. Cook for an additional 10-15 minutes until the quinoa is cooked, and the kale is tender.

6. Season the minestrone with salt and pepper to taste. Take out the bay leaf.

7. Ladle the minestrone into bowls and garnish with fresh parsley. Serve with vegan Parmesan on the side if desired.

Nutritional Information (per serving):

- **Carbs:** 40g
- **Fats:** 5g
- **Fiber:** 8g
- **Protein:** 10g

Chapter 4: Salads

Quinoa and Avocado Anti-Inflammatory Salad

Prep Time: 15 minutes | Cook Time: 15 minutes | Servings: 4

Ingredients:

- 1 cup quinoa, rinsed and drained
- 2 cups water
- 1 cup cherry tomatoes, halved
- 1 cucumber, diced
- 1 red bell pepper, diced
- 1/4 cup red onion, finely chopped
- 1/4 cup fresh cilantro, chopped
- 2 ripe avocados, diced
- Juice of 2 limes
- 3 tablespoons extra-virgin olive oil
- 1 teaspoon ground turmeric
- 1 teaspoon ground ginger
- Salt and pepper to taste

Instructions:

1. In a medium-sized saucepan, put together the quinoa and water. Bring to a boil, then reduce heat to low, cover, and simmer for 15 minutes, or until the quinoa is cooked and water is absorbed.

2. While the quinoa is cooking, prepare the vegetables. In a large bowl, put together the cherry tomatoes, cucumber, red bell pepper, red onion, and cilantro.

3. In a small bowl, whisk together the lime juice, extra-virgin olive oil, ground turmeric, ground ginger, salt, and pepper to create the dressing.

4. Once the quinoa is cooked, fluff it with a fork and let it cool for a few minutes.

5. Add the cooled quinoa and diced avocados to the bowl with the vegetables.

6. Pour the dressing over the salad and gently toss until all ingredients are well coated.

7. Serve immediately or refrigerate for later.

Nutritional Information (per serving):

- Carbs: 45g
- Fats: 20g
- Fiber: 11g
- Protein: 8g

Cucumber Mint Detox Salad

Prep Time: 20 minutes | Cook Time: 0 minutes | Servings: 4

Ingredients:

- 2 large cucumbers, thinly sliced
- 1 cup cherry tomatoes, halved
- 1/2 red onion, thinly sliced
- 1/4 cup fresh mint leaves, chopped
- 1 avocado, diced
- 1/4 cup pumpkin seeds
- Juice of 1 lemon
- 3 tablespoons extra-virgin olive oil
- 1 teaspoon ground cumin
- Salt and pepper to taste

Instructions:

1. In a large bowl, put together the thinly sliced cucumbers, cherry tomatoes, red onion, chopped mint leaves, diced avocado, and pumpkin seeds.

2. In a small bowl, whisk together the lemon juice, extra-virgin olive oil, ground cumin, salt, and pepper to create the dressing.

3. Pour the dressing over the salad and toss gently to ensure even coating.

4. Allow the salad to marinate for at least 10 minutes to enhance the flavors.

5. Serve chilled and enjoy your refreshing Cucumber Mint Detox Salad!

Nutritional Information (per serving):

- Carbs: 18g
- Fats: 14g
- Fiber: 7g
- Protein: 4g

Roasted Beet and Walnut Arugula Salad

Prep Time: 15 minutes | Cook Time: 45 minutes | Servings: 4

Ingredients:

- 4 medium-sized beets, peeled and diced
- 1 cup walnuts, chopped
- 6 cups arugula
- 1/2 red onion, thinly sliced
- 1/4 cup fresh parsley, chopped
- 1/4 cup balsamic vinegar
- 3 tablespoons extra-virgin olive oil
- 1 tablespoon maple syrup
- Salt and pepper to taste

Instructions:

1. Preheat the oven to 400°F (200°C).

2. Place the diced beets on a baking sheet, drizzle with olive oil, and season with salt and pepper. Roast in the preheated oven for about 45 minutes or until the beets are tender and slightly caramelized.

3. While the beets are roasting, toast the chopped walnuts in a dry skillet over medium heat until they become fragrant. Stir frequently to prevent burning. Set aside.

4. In a large salad bowl, put together the arugula, thinly sliced red onion, and chopped parsley.

5. In a small bowl, whisk together the balsamic vinegar, extra-virgin olive oil, maple syrup, salt, and pepper to create the dressing.

6. Once the beets are roasted, let them cool for a few minutes, then add them to the salad bowl.

7. Drizzle the dressing over the salad and toss gently to combine all ingredients.

8. Top the salad with the toasted walnuts.

9. Serve immediately and enjoy your delicious Roasted Beet and Walnut Arugula Salad!

Nutritional Information (per serving):

- Carbs: 28g
- Fats: 19g
- Fiber: 7g
- Protein: 5g

Turmeric Tahini Kale Salad

Prep Time: 15 minutes | Cook Time: 0 minutes | Servings: 4

Ingredients:

- 1 bunch kale, stems removed, and leaves finely chopped
- 1 cup cherry tomatoes, halved
- 1 cucumber, thinly sliced
- 1/4 cup red onion, finely chopped
- 1/4 cup sunflower seeds
- 1/4 cup raisins
- 1/4 cup fresh cilantro, chopped

Turmeric Tahini Dressing:

- 1/4 cup tahini
- 2 tablespoons extra-virgin olive oil
- Juice of 1 lemon
- 1 teaspoon ground turmeric
- 1 clove garlic, minced
- Salt and pepper to taste

Instructions:

1. In a large salad bowl, put together the finely chopped kale, cherry tomatoes, thinly sliced cucumber, finely chopped red onion, sunflower seeds, raisins, and chopped cilantro.

2. In a separate small bowl, whisk together the tahini, extra-virgin olive oil, lemon juice, ground turmeric, minced garlic, salt, and pepper to create the Turmeric Tahini Dressing.

3. Pour the dressing over the kale salad.

4. Using your hands, massage the dressing into the kale leaves for a few minutes. This helps to soften the kale and allows it to absorb the flavors.

5. Let the salad sit for at least 10 minutes to marinate and enhance the flavors.

6. Serve chilled, and enjoy your vibrant and nutritious Turmeric Tahini Kale Salad!

Nutritional Information (per serving):

- Carbs: 24g
- Fats: 18g
- Fiber: 5g
- Protein: 7g

Blueberry Almond Spinach Salad

Prep Time: 10 minutes | Cook Time: 0 minutes | Servings: 4

Ingredients:

- 6 cups fresh spinach leaves, washed and dried
- 1 cup blueberries, washed
- 1/2 cup sliced almonds, toasted
- 1/4 cup red onion, thinly sliced
- 1/4 cup fresh basil leaves, chopped

Lemon Poppy Seed Dressing:

- 3 tablespoons extra-virgin olive oil
- Juice of 1 lemon
- 1 tablespoon maple syrup
- 1 teaspoon Dijon mustard
- 1 teaspoon poppy seeds
- Salt and pepper to taste

Instructions:

1. In a large salad bowl, put together the fresh spinach leaves, washed blueberries, toasted sliced almonds, thinly sliced red onion, and chopped fresh basil leaves.

2. In a small bowl, whisk together the extra-virgin olive oil, lemon juice, maple syrup, Dijon mustard, poppy seeds, salt, and pepper to create the Lemon Poppy Seed Dressing.

3. Pour the dressing over the spinach salad.

4. Toss the salad gently to ensure even coating with the dressing.

5. Serve immediately for optimal freshness.

Nutritional Information (per serving):

- Carbs: 18g
- Fats: 14g
- Fiber: 6g
- Protein: 4g

Mango Basil Summer Salad

Prep Time: 15 minutes | Cook Time: 0 minutes | Servings: 4

Ingredients:

- 4 cups mixed salad greens
- 2 ripe mangoes, peeled and diced
- 1 cup cherry tomatoes, halved
- 1 cucumber, thinly sliced
- 1/4 cup red onion, finely chopped
- 1/4 cup fresh basil leaves, torn
- 1/4 cup pine nuts, toasted

Citrus Vinaigrette:

- 3 tablespoons extra-virgin olive oil
- Juice of 1 orange
- Juice of 1 lime
- 1 teaspoon agave syrup or maple syrup
- Salt and pepper to taste

Instructions:

1. In a large salad bowl, put together the mixed salad greens, diced mangoes, halved cherry tomatoes, thinly sliced cucumber, finely chopped red onion, torn fresh basil leaves, and toasted pine nuts.

2. In a small bowl, whisk together the extra-virgin olive oil, orange juice, lime juice, agave syrup (or maple syrup), salt, and pepper to create the Citrus Vinaigrette.

3. Pour the vinaigrette over the mango salad.

4. Gently toss the salad to ensure all ingredients are well coated with the vinaigrette.

5. Serve immediately to enjoy the freshness of the Mango Basil Summer Salad.

Nutritional Information (per serving):

- Carbs: 26g
- Fats: 14g
- Fiber: 5g
- Protein: 3g

Roasted Brussels Sprouts and Pomegranate Salad

Prep Time: 15 minutes | Cook Time: 25 minutes | Servings: 4

Ingredients:

- 1 lb Brussels sprouts, trimmed and halved
- 1 tablespoon olive oil
- Salt and pepper to taste
- 1 cup pomegranate arils
- 1/2 cup pecans, toasted and chopped
- 4 cups mixed salad greens
- 1/4 cup red onion, thinly sliced
- 1/4 cup balsamic vinegar
- 3 tablespoons extra-virgin olive oil
- 1 tablespoon maple syrup
- 1 teaspoon Dijon mustard

Instructions:

1. Preheat the oven to 400°F (200°C).

2. In a large mixing bowl, toss the halved Brussels sprouts with olive oil, salt, and pepper until evenly coated. Spread them on a baking sheet in a single layer.

3. Roast the Brussels sprouts in the preheated oven for about 25 minutes or until they are golden brown and crispy on the edges. Remove from the oven and let them cool slightly.

4. In a small bowl, whisk together the balsamic vinegar, extra-virgin olive oil, maple syrup, and Dijon mustard to create the dressing.

5. In a large salad bowl, put together the roasted Brussels sprouts, pomegranate arils, toasted and chopped pecans, mixed salad greens, and thinly sliced red onion.

6. Drizzle the dressing over the salad and toss gently to coat all the ingredients.

7. Serve the Roasted Brussels Sprouts and Pomegranate Salad immediately to enjoy the flavors and textures.

Nutritional Information (per serving):

- Carbs: 29g
- Fats: 18g
- Fiber: 7g
- Protein: 5g

<u>Asparagus and Almond Quinoa Salad</u>

Prep Time: 15 minutes | Cook Time: 15 minutes | Servings: 4

Ingredients:

- 1 cup quinoa, rinsed and drained
- 2 cups water
- 1 bunch asparagus, ends trimmed and cut into 2-inch pieces
- 1/2 cup almonds, sliced and toasted
- 1 red bell pepper, diced
- 1/4 cup fresh parsley, chopped
- 1/4 cup green onions, thinly sliced
- 3 tablespoons extra-virgin olive oil
- Juice of 1 lemon
- 1 teaspoon Dijon mustard
- Salt and pepper to taste

Instructions:

1. In a medium-sized saucepan, put together the quinoa and water. Bring to a boil, then reduce heat to low, cover, and simmer for 15 minutes, or until the quinoa is cooked and water is absorbed.

2. While the quinoa is cooking, steam the asparagus for 3-5 minutes until tender-crisp. Alternatively, you can blanch them in boiling water for 2-3 minutes. Drain and set aside.

3. In a large salad bowl, put together the cooked quinoa, steamed asparagus, sliced and toasted almonds, diced red bell pepper, chopped fresh parsley, and thinly sliced green onions.

4. In a small bowl, whisk together the extra-virgin olive oil, lemon juice, Dijon mustard, salt, and pepper to create the dressing.

5. Pour the dressing over the quinoa salad and toss gently to combine all ingredients.

6. Serve the Asparagus and Almond Quinoa Salad at room temperature or chilled.

Nutritional Information (per serving):

- Carbs: 36g
- Fats: 17g
- Fiber: 7g
- Protein: 9g

Turmeric Mango Cilantro Slaw

Prep Time: 20 minutes | Cook Time: 0 minutes | Servings: 4

Ingredients:

- 1 small green cabbage, thinly shredded
- 1 large carrot, julienned
- 1 ripe mango, peeled and julienned
- 1/4 cup fresh cilantro, chopped
- 1/4 cup red onion, thinly sliced
- 1/4 cup pepitas (pumpkin seeds), toasted

Turmeric Mango Dressing:

- 3 tablespoons extra-virgin olive oil
- Juice of 2 limes
- 1 teaspoon ground turmeric
- 1 teaspoon agave syrup or maple syrup
- Salt and pepper to taste

Instructions:

1. In a large mixing bowl, put together the thinly shredded green cabbage, julienned carrot, julienned mango, chopped fresh cilantro, thinly sliced red onion, and toasted pepitas.

2. In a small bowl, whisk together the extra-virgin olive oil, lime juice, ground turmeric, agave syrup (or maple syrup), salt, and pepper to create the Turmeric Mango Dressing.

3. Pour the dressing over the slaw and toss gently to ensure all ingredients are well coated.

4. Allow the Turmeric Mango Cilantro Slaw to sit for about 10 minutes to let the flavors meld.

5. Serve the slaw chilled or at room temperature.

Nutritional Information (per serving):

- Carbs: 22g
- Fats: 12g
- Fiber: 5g
- Protein: 4g

Mediterranean Lentil and Artichoke Salad
Prep Time: 15 minutes | Cook Time: 20 minutes | Servings: 4

Ingredients:

- 1 cup dry green lentils, rinsed and drained
- 2 1/2 cups water
- 1 can (14 oz) artichoke hearts, drained and quartered
- 1 cup cherry tomatoes, halved
- 1/2 cup cucumber, diced
- 1/4 cup red onion, finely chopped
- 1/4 cup Kalamata olives, sliced
- 1/4 cup fresh parsley, chopped
- 1/4 cup extra-virgin olive oil
- Juice of 1 lemon
- 2 cloves garlic, minced
- 1 teaspoon dried oregano
- Salt and pepper to taste

Instructions:

1. In a medium-sized saucepan, put together the rinsed green lentils and water. Bring to a boil, then reduce heat to low, cover, and simmer for 20 minutes or until the lentils are tender. Drain any excess water.

2. In a large salad bowl, put together the cooked lentils, quartered artichoke hearts, halved cherry tomatoes, diced cucumber, finely chopped red onion, sliced Kalamata olives, and chopped fresh parsley.

3. In a small bowl, whisk together the extra-virgin olive oil, lemon juice, minced garlic, dried oregano, salt, and pepper to create the dressing.

4. Pour the dressing over the lentil and artichoke mixture.

5. Toss the salad gently to ensure all ingredients are well coated with the dressing.

6. Allow the Mediterranean Lentil and Artichoke Salad to marinate for at least 15 minutes to enhance the flavors.

7. Serve the salad chilled or at room temperature.

Nutritional Information (per serving):

- Carbs: 35g
- Fats: 14g
- Fiber: 12g
- Protein: 12g

Watermelon Basil Arugula Salad

Prep Time: 15 minutes | Cook Time: 0 minutes | Servings: 4

Ingredients:

- 4 cups arugula, washed and dried
- 2 cups watermelon, diced
- 1/2 cup red onion, thinly sliced
- 1/4 cup fresh basil leaves, torn
- 1/4 cup vegan feta cheese, crumbled (optional)
- 1/4 cup balsamic vinegar
- 3 tablespoons extra-virgin olive oil
- Salt and pepper to taste

Instructions:

1. In a large salad bowl, put together the washed and dried arugula, diced watermelon, thinly sliced red onion, torn fresh basil leaves, and crumbled vegan feta cheese (if using).

2. In a small bowl, whisk together the balsamic vinegar, extra-virgin olive oil, salt, and pepper to create the dressing.

3. Pour the dressing over the Watermelon Basil Arugula Salad.

4. Toss the salad gently to ensure all ingredients are well coated with the dressing.

5. Serve the salad immediately to enjoy the crispness and freshness.

Nutritional Information (per serving):

- Carbs: 18g
- Fats: 11g
- Fiber: 2g
- Protein: 2g

<u>Orange Fennel Detox Salad</u>

Prep Time: 20 minutes | Cook Time: 0 minutes | Servings: 4

Ingredients:

- 1 large fennel bulb, thinly sliced
- 2 oranges, peeled and segmented
- 1 avocado, diced
- 1/4 cup red onion, thinly sliced
- 1/4 cup fresh mint leaves, chopped
- 1/4 cup pomegranate arils
- 1/4 cup slivered almonds, toasted

Citrus Detox Dressing:

- 3 tablespoons extra-virgin olive oil
- Juice of 2 oranges
- Juice of 1 lemon
- 1 teaspoon agave syrup or maple syrup
- 1/2 teaspoon ground turmeric
- Salt and pepper to taste

Instructions:

1. In a large salad bowl, put together the thinly sliced fennel bulb, peeled and segmented oranges, diced avocado, thinly sliced red onion, chopped fresh mint leaves, pomegranate arils, and toasted slivered almonds.

2. In a small bowl, whisk together the extra-virgin olive oil, orange juice, lemon juice, agave syrup (or maple syrup), ground turmeric, salt, and pepper to create the Citrus Detox Dressing.

3. Pour the dressing over the Orange Fennel Detox Salad.

4. Toss the salad gently to ensure all ingredients are well coated with the detox dressing.

5. Allow the salad to marinate for at least 10 minutes to enhance the flavors.

6. Serve the detox salad chilled and enjoy the revitalizing combination of flavors.

Nutritional Information (per serving):

- Carbs: 26g
- Fats: 16g
- Fiber: 8g
- Protein: 4g

Avocado Tomato Basil Detox Salad

Prep Time: 15 minutes | Cook Time: 0 minutes | Servings: 4

Ingredients:

- 4 cups mixed salad greens
- 2 avocados, diced
- 2 cups cherry tomatoes, halved
- 1/4 cup red onion, finely chopped
- 1/4 cup fresh basil leaves, torn
- 1/4 cup sunflower seeds, toasted

Detox Lemon-Garlic Dressing:

- 3 tablespoons extra-virgin olive oil
- Juice of 1 lemon
- 2 cloves garlic, minced
- 1 teaspoon agave syrup or maple syrup
- Salt and pepper to taste

Instructions:

1. In a large salad bowl, put together the mixed salad greens, diced avocados, halved cherry tomatoes, finely chopped red onion, torn fresh basil leaves, and toasted sunflower seeds.

2. In a small bowl, whisk together the extra-virgin olive oil, lemon juice, minced garlic, agave syrup (or maple syrup), salt, and pepper to create the Detox Lemon-Garlic Dressing.

3. Pour the dressing over the Avocado Tomato Basil Detox Salad.

4. Toss the salad gently to ensure all ingredients are well coated with the detox dressing.

5. Allow the salad to marinate for at least 10 minutes to enhance the flavors.

6. Serve the detox salad chilled and savor the vibrant and nourishing combination.

Nutritional Information (per serving):

- Carbs: 19g
- Fats: 17g
- Fiber: 8g
- Protein: 4g

Roasted Cauliflower and Cumin Chickpea Salad

Prep Time: 15 minutes | Cook Time: 30 minutes | Servings: 4

Ingredients:

- 1 head cauliflower, cut into florets
- 1 can (15 oz) chickpeas, drained and rinsed
- 3 tablespoons olive oil
- 2 teaspoons ground cumin
- Salt and pepper to taste
- 4 cups mixed salad greens
- 1/4 cup red onion, finely sliced
- 1/4 cup fresh parsley, chopped
- 1/4 cup lemon juice
- 3 tablespoons tahini
- 2 cloves garlic, minced
- 1 teaspoon agave syrup or maple syrup

Instructions:

1. Preheat the oven to 400°F (200°C).

2. In a large mixing bowl, toss the cauliflower florets and chickpeas with olive oil, ground cumin, salt, and pepper until evenly coated.

3. Spread the cauliflower and chickpea mixture on a baking sheet in a single layer.

4. Roast in the preheated oven for about 30 minutes or until the cauliflower is golden brown and chickpeas are crispy. Stir halfway through for even roasting.

5. In a large salad bowl, put together the mixed salad greens, finely sliced red onion, and chopped fresh parsley.

6. In a small bowl, whisk together the lemon juice, tahini, minced garlic, agave syrup (or maple syrup), salt, and pepper to create the dressing.

7. Once the roasted cauliflower and chickpeas are done, let them cool slightly before adding them to the salad bowl.

8. Pour the tahini dressing over the salad and toss gently to ensure all ingredients are well coated.

9. Serve the Roasted Cauliflower and Cumin Chickpea Salad warm or at room temperature.

Nutritional Information (per serving):

- Carbs: 35g
- Fats: 18g
- Fiber: 10g
- Protein: 11g

Arugula Pomegranate Quinoa Salad

Prep Time: 20 minutes | Cook Time: 15 minutes | Servings: 4

Ingredients:

- 1 cup quinoa, rinsed and drained
- 2 cups water
- 4 cups arugula, washed and dried
- 1 cup pomegranate arils
- 1/2 cup walnuts, chopped and toasted
- 1/4 cup red onion, finely sliced
- 1/4 cup fresh mint leaves, chopped

Balsamic Dijon Dressing:

- 3 tablespoons extra-virgin olive oil
- 2 tablespoons balsamic vinegar
- 1 tablespoon Dijon mustard
- 1 clove garlic, minced
- Salt and pepper to taste

Instructions:

1. In a medium-sized saucepan, put together the rinsed quinoa and water. Bring to a boil, then reduce heat to low, cover, and simmer for 15 minutes or until the quinoa is cooked and water is absorbed. Fluff with a fork and let it cool.

2. In a large salad bowl, put together the cooked quinoa, arugula, pomegranate arils, toasted chopped walnuts, finely sliced red onion, and chopped fresh mint leaves.

3. In a small bowl, whisk together the extra-virgin olive oil, balsamic vinegar, Dijon mustard, minced garlic, salt, and pepper to create the Balsamic Dijon Dressing.

4. Pour the dressing over the Arugula Pomegranate Quinoa Salad.

5. Toss the salad gently to ensure all ingredients are well coated with the dressing.

6. Allow the salad to sit for a few minutes to let the flavors meld.

7. Serve the quinoa salad at room temperature or chilled.

Nutritional Information (per serving):

- Carbs: 39g
- Fats: 16g
- Fiber: 6g
- Protein: 8g

Turmeric Roasted Carrot and Chickpea Salad

Prep Time: 15 minutes | Cook Time: 25 minutes | Servings: 4

Ingredients:

- 1 lb carrots, peeled and sliced into sticks
- 1 can (15 oz) chickpeas, drained and rinsed
- 3 tablespoons olive oil
- 1 teaspoon ground turmeric
- 1 teaspoon ground cumin
- 1 teaspoon smoked paprika
- Salt and pepper to taste
- 4 cups mixed salad greens
- 1/4 cup red onion, finely sliced
- 1/4 cup fresh cilantro, chopped

Tahini Lemon Dressing:

- 3 tablespoons tahini
- Juice of 1 lemon
- 2 tablespoons water
- 1 clove garlic, minced
- Salt and pepper to taste

Instructions:

1. Preheat the oven to 400°F (200°C).

2. In a large mixing bowl, toss the sliced carrots and chickpeas with olive oil, ground turmeric, ground cumin, smoked paprika, salt, and pepper until well coated.

3. Spread the seasoned carrots and chickpeas on a baking sheet in a single layer.

4. Roast in the preheated oven for about 25 minutes or until the carrots are tender and chickpeas are crispy. Stir halfway through for even roasting.

5. In a large salad bowl, put together the mixed salad greens, finely sliced red onion, and chopped fresh cilantro.

6. In a small bowl, whisk together the tahini, lemon juice, water, minced garlic, salt, and pepper to create the Tahini Lemon Dressing.

7. Once the roasted carrots and chickpeas are done, let them cool slightly before adding them to the salad bowl.

8. Pour the tahini lemon dressing over the salad and toss gently to ensure all ingredients are well coated.

9. Serve the Turmeric Roasted Carrot and Chickpea Salad warm or at room temperature.

Nutritional Information (per serving):

Carbs: 35g | Fats: 17g | Fiber: 10g | Protein: 9g

Mango Avocado Black Bean Salad

Prep Time: 20 minutes | Cook Time: 0 minutes | Servings: 4

Ingredients:

- 1 can (15 oz) black beans, drained and rinsed
- 2 ripe mangoes, peeled and diced
- 2 avocados, diced
- 1/2 cup red onion, finely chopped
- 1/4 cup fresh cilantro, chopped
- 1 jalapeño, seeds removed and finely chopped (optional)
- Juice of 2 limes
- 3 tablespoons extra-virgin olive oil
- Salt and pepper to taste
- 4 cups mixed salad greens

Instructions:

1. In a large salad bowl, put together the black beans, diced mangoes, diced avocados, finely chopped red onion, chopped fresh cilantro, and finely chopped jalapeño (if using).
2. Squeeze the juice of 2 limes over the salad ingredients.
3. Drizzle the extra-virgin olive oil over the salad.
4. Season the Mango Avocado Black Bean Salad with salt and pepper to taste.
5. Gently toss the salad to ensure all ingredients are well combined.
6. Serve the salad over a bed of mixed salad greens.

Nutritional Information (per serving):

- Carbs: 50g
- Fats: 22g
- Fiber: 16g
- Protein: 12g

Spinach Strawberry Walnut Salad with Balsamic Vinaigrette

Prep Time: 15 minutes | Cook Time: 0 minutes | Servings: 4

Ingredients:

- 8 cups fresh baby spinach, washed and dried
- 2 cups strawberries, hulled and sliced
- 1 cup walnuts, chopped and toasted
- 1/2 cup red onion, thinly sliced
- 1/4 cup fresh basil leaves, torn

Balsamic Vinaigrette:

- 1/3 cup extra-virgin olive oil
- 1/4 cup balsamic vinegar
- 1 tablespoon Dijon mustard
- 1 clove garlic, minced
- Salt and pepper to taste

Instructions:

1. In a large salad bowl, put together the fresh baby spinach, sliced strawberries, toasted chopped walnuts, thinly sliced red onion, and torn fresh basil leaves.
2. In a small bowl, whisk together the extra-virgin olive oil, balsamic vinegar, Dijon mustard, minced garlic, salt, and pepper to create the Balsamic Vinaigrette.
3. Pour the Balsamic Vinaigrette over the Spinach Strawberry Walnut Salad.
4. Toss the salad gently to ensure all ingredients are well coated with the vinaigrette.
5. Allow the salad to sit for a few minutes to let the flavors meld.
6. Serve the Spinach Strawberry Walnut Salad immediately and enjoy the delightful combination of flavors and textures.

Nutritional Information (per serving):

- Carbs: 19g
- Fats: 26g
- Fiber: 7g
- Protein: 5g

49

Chapter 5: Main Courses

Eggplant and Chickpea Turmeric Curry

Prep Time: 15 minutes | **Cook Time:** 30 minutes | **Number of Servings:** 4

Ingredients:

- 1 cup dried chickpeas, soaked overnight
- 2 eggplants, diced
- 1 large onion, finely chopped
- 3 cloves garlic, minced
- 1-inch fresh ginger, grated
- 1 can (400g) diced tomatoes
- 1 can (400ml) coconut milk
- 2 teaspoons ground turmeric
- 1 teaspoon ground cumin
- 1 teaspoon ground coriander
- 1 teaspoon paprika
- 1/2 teaspoon cinnamon
- 1/4 teaspoon cayenne pepper
- 2 tablespoons olive oil
- Salt and pepper to taste
- Fresh cilantro for garnish

Instructions:

1. Drain and rinse the soaked chickpeas. In a pot, cover them with water and simmer until tender, approximately 20-25 minutes. Drain and set aside.

2. In a large pan, heat olive oil over medium heat. Add chopped onions, minced garlic, and grated ginger. Sauté until the onions are soft and translucent.

3. Stir in ground turmeric, ground cumin, ground coriander, paprika, cinnamon, and cayenne pepper. Cook for an additional 2 minutes to toast the spices.

4. Add diced eggplants to the pan and cook until they start to soften.

5. Pour in the diced tomatoes and coconut milk. Stir adequately to combine all the ingredients.

6. Bring the mixture to a simmer and let it cook for about 15-20 minutes, allowing the flavors to meld and the curry to thicken.

7. Incorporate the cooked chickpeas into the curry. Cook for an additional 5-7 minutes until the chickpeas are heated through.

8. Season with salt and pepper to taste. Adjust the spices if necessary.

9. Garnish the curry with fresh cilantro before serving.

Nutritional Information (per serving):

Carbs: 45g | **Fats:** 15g | **Fiber:** 12g | **Protein:** 10g

Lentil and Vegetable Stir-Fry

Prep Time: 20 minutes | **Cook Time:** 15 minutes | **Number of Servings:** 4

Ingredients:

- 1 cup dried green lentils, cooked
- 2 cups broccoli florets
- 1 red bell pepper, thinly sliced
- 1 yellow bell pepper, thinly sliced
- 1 medium carrot, julienned
- 1 cup snap peas, trimmed
- 4 green onions, sliced
- 3 cloves garlic, minced
- 1-inch fresh ginger, julienned
- 1/4 cup tamari (gluten-free soy sauce)
- 2 tablespoons sesame oil
- 1 tablespoon maple syrup
- 1 tablespoon rice vinegar
- 1 teaspoon sriracha sauce (optional)
- 2 tablespoons sesame seeds for garnish
- Fresh cilantro for garnish

Instructions:

1. Cook the dried green lentils according to package instructions. Drain and set aside.

2. Cut broccoli into small florets, thinly slice the red and yellow bell peppers, julienne the carrot, trim snap peas, slice green onions, mince garlic, and julienne fresh ginger.

3. Heat sesame oil in a large wok or pan over medium-high heat. Add sliced bell peppers, broccoli florets, julienned carrots, and snap peas. Stir-fry for 4-5 minutes until the vegetables are tender-crisp.

4. Add minced garlic and julienned ginger to the vegetables. Stir-fry for an additional 1-2 minutes until fragrant.

5. Add the cooked green lentils to the vegetable mixture. Stir adequately to combine.

6. In a small bowl, whisk together tamari, maple syrup, rice vinegar, and sriracha sauce (if using).

7. Pour the sauce over the lentil and vegetable mixture. Toss everything together until evenly coated and heated through.

8. Taste and adjust the seasoning, adding more tamari or maple syrup if needed.

9. Garnish the stir-fry with sesame seeds and fresh cilantro.

Nutritional Information (per serving):

Carbs: 40g | **Fats:** 8g | **Fiber:** 12g | **Protein:** 15g

Spaghetti Squash with Roasted Tomato Sauce

Prep Time: 15 minutes | **Cook Time:** 45 minutes | **Number of Servings:** 4

Ingredients:

- 2 medium spaghetti squash, halved and seeds removed
- 1.5 lbs cherry tomatoes
- 3 cloves garlic, minced
- 1 small red onion, finely chopped
- 2 tablespoons olive oil
- 1 teaspoon dried oregano
- 1 teaspoon dried basil
- 1/2 teaspoon red pepper flakes (optional)
- Salt and pepper to taste
- Fresh basil leaves for garnish

Instructions:

1. Preheat the oven to 400°F (200°C).

2. Place the halved spaghetti squash on a baking sheet, cut side up. Roast in the preheated oven for 40-45 minutes or until the squash is fork-tender.

3. On a separate baking sheet, toss cherry tomatoes with olive oil, minced garlic, dried oregano, dried basil, red pepper flakes (if using), salt, and pepper. Roast in the oven for 20-25 minutes or until tomatoes are blistered and caramelized.

4. In a pan, sauté the finely chopped red onion in olive oil until it becomes translucent and slightly caramelized.

5. Once the tomatoes are roasted, transfer them to the pan with sautéed onions. Mash the tomatoes with a fork or potato masher to create a chunky sauce. Simmer for an additional 5-10 minutes to meld the flavors.

6. Scrape the roasted spaghetti squash with a fork to create "spaghetti" strands. Place them in a serving dish.

7. Pour the roasted tomato sauce over the spaghetti squash strands. Toss gently to coat the squash with the sauce.

8. Garnish with fresh basil leaves before serving.

Nutritional Information (per serving):

- **Carbs:** 30g
- **Fats:** 8g
- **Fiber:** 8g
- **Protein:** 3g

Quinoa-Stuffed Portobello Mushrooms

Prep Time: 20 minutes | **Cook Time:** 25 minutes | **Number of Servings:** 4

Ingredients:

- 4 large portobello mushrooms, stems removed
- 1 cup quinoa, rinsed
- 2 cups vegetable broth
- 1 small red onion, finely diced
- 2 cloves garlic, minced
- 1 red bell pepper, finely diced
- 1 zucchini, diced
- 1 cup cherry tomatoes, halved
- 1/4 cup pine nuts
- 1 teaspoon dried thyme
- 1 teaspoon dried rosemary
- 1/2 teaspoon smoked paprika
- 2 tablespoons olive oil
- Salt and pepper to taste
- Fresh parsley for garnish

Instructions:

1. Preheat the oven to 375°F (190°C).

2. Clean the portobello mushrooms and take out the stems. Place them on a baking sheet, gill side up.

3. In a saucepan, combine quinoa and vegetable broth. Bring to a boil, then reduce heat to low, cover, and simmer for 15 minutes or until the quinoa is cooked and liquid is absorbed.

4. In a pan, heat olive oil over medium heat. Add finely diced red onion, minced garlic, and diced zucchini. Sauté until the vegetables are softened.

5. Add finely diced red bell pepper and halved cherry tomatoes to the pan. Cook for an additional 3-5 minutes until the vegetables are tender.

6. Stir in pine nuts, dried thyme, dried rosemary, smoked paprika, salt, and pepper. Toast the pine nuts until they are golden brown and fragrant.

7. Add the cooked quinoa to the pan with sautéed vegetables and mix adequately to combine.

8. Fill each portobello mushroom cap with the quinoa and vegetable mixture.

9. Bake in the preheated oven for 20-25 minutes or until the mushrooms are tender.

10. Garnish with fresh parsley before serving.

Nutritional Information (per serving):

Carbs: 35g | **Fats:** 12g | **Fiber:** 7g | **Protein:** 9g

Coconut Turmeric Tofu Skewers

Prep Time: 30 minutes | **Cook Time:** 15 minutes | **Number of Servings:** 4

Ingredients:

- 1 block (14 oz) extra-firm tofu, pressed and cubed
- 1 can (400ml) coconut milk
- 2 tablespoons tamari (gluten-free soy sauce)
- 1 tablespoon maple syrup
- 1 tablespoon lime juice
- 1 tablespoon turmeric powder
- 2 teaspoons curry powder
- 1 teaspoon cumin
- 1 teaspoon paprika
- 1 teaspoon garlic powder
- 1 red bell pepper, diced
- 1 yellow bell pepper, diced
- 1 zucchini, sliced
- 1 red onion, sliced into chunks
- Wooden skewers, soaked in water

Instructions:

1. Press the tofu to remove excess water, then cut it into cubes.

2. In a bowl, combine coconut milk, tamari, maple syrup, lime juice, turmeric powder, curry powder, cumin, paprika, and garlic powder. Mix adequately to create the marinade.

3. Place tofu cubes in a shallow dish and pour half of the marinade over them. Allow the tofu to marinate for at least 15-20 minutes.

4. In the meantime, dice red and yellow bell peppers, slice zucchini, and cut the red onion into chunks.

5. Thread marinated tofu cubes, diced bell peppers, sliced zucchini, and red onion chunks onto soaked wooden skewers.

6. Grill the skewers on a barbecue or grill pan for about 12-15 minutes, turning occasionally until the tofu and vegetables are cooked and have a nice char. Alternatively, you can bake them in the oven at 400°F (200°C) for the same duration.

7. While grilling or baking, baste the skewers with the remaining marinade to enhance the flavor.

8. Once cooked, take out the skewers from the grill or oven. Serve immediately.

Nutritional Information (per serving):

- **Carbs:** 20g
- **Fats:** 18g
- **Fiber:** 4g
- **Protein:** 15g

Zucchini Noodles with Creamy Avocado Pesto

Prep Time: 15 minutes | **Cook Time:** 0 minutes | **Number of Servings:** 4

Ingredients:

- 4 medium zucchinis, spiralized into noodles
- 2 ripe avocados, peeled and pitted
- 1 cup fresh basil leaves
- 1/2 cup fresh parsley leaves
- 3 cloves garlic, minced
- 1/4 cup pine nuts
- 1/4 cup nutritional yeast
- 2 tablespoons lemon juice
- 3 tablespoons olive oil
- Salt and pepper to taste
- Cherry tomatoes for garnish (optional)
- Hemp seeds for garnish (optional)

Instructions:

1. Spiralize the zucchinis into noodles and set aside.

2. In a food processor, combine ripe avocados, fresh basil leaves, fresh parsley leaves, minced garlic, pine nuts, nutritional yeast, lemon juice, olive oil, salt, and pepper. Blend until smooth and creamy.

3. Pour the creamy avocado pesto over the zucchini noodles. Toss until the noodles are evenly coated with the pesto.

4. Garnish the zucchini noodles with cherry tomatoes and hemp seeds if desired.

5. Serve immediately, and enjoy the refreshing and creamy zucchini noodle dish.

Nutritional Information (per serving):

- **Carbs:** 15g
- **Fats:** 20g
- **Fiber:** 10g
- **Protein:** 5g

Sesame Crusted Tofu with Turmeric Citrus Glaze

Prep Time: 30 minutes | **Cook Time:** 15 minutes | **Number of Servings:** 4

Ingredients:

For Sesame Crusted Tofu:

- 1 block (14 oz) extra-firm tofu, pressed and sliced into rectangles
- 1/2 cup sesame seeds
- 1/4 cup tamari (gluten-free soy sauce)
- 1 tablespoon rice vinegar
- 1 tablespoon sesame oil
- 1 teaspoon ginger, grated
- 1 teaspoon garlic powder
- 2 tablespoons cornstarch

For Turmeric Citrus Glaze:

- 1/4 cup orange juice
- 2 tablespoons maple syrup
- 1 teaspoon turmeric powder
- 1 teaspoon lime juice
- 1/2 teaspoon orange zest
- Salt and pepper to taste

Instructions:

1. Press the tofu to remove excess water, then slice it into rectangles.

2. In a bowl, combine tamari, rice vinegar, sesame oil, grated ginger, and garlic powder. Marinate the tofu slices in this mixture for at least 15-20 minutes.

3. In a separate bowl, mix sesame seeds and cornstarch. Coat each tofu slice with the sesame seed mixture, pressing the seeds onto the tofu.

4. Heat a pan over medium heat. Pan-fry the sesame-crusted tofu slices until golden brown and crispy on both sides.

5. In a small saucepan, combine orange juice, maple syrup, turmeric powder, lime juice, orange zest, salt, and pepper. Simmer over low heat until the glaze thickens slightly.

6. Pour the turmeric citrus glaze over the pan-fried tofu slices, ensuring they are evenly coated. Allow the glaze to heat through for an additional 2-3 minutes.

7. Serve the sesame-crusted tofu with turmeric citrus glaze immediately.

Nutritional Information (per serving):

Carbs: 15g | **Fats:** 12g | **Fiber:** 3g | **Protein:** 10g

Portobello Mushroom and Spinach Stuffed Peppers

Prep Time: 25 minutes | **Cook Time:** 30 minutes | **Number of Servings:** 4

Ingredients:

- 4 large bell peppers, halved and seeds removed
- 2 cups baby spinach, chopped
- 4 large portobello mushrooms, diced
- 1 cup quinoa, cooked
- 1 can (15 oz) black beans, drained and rinsed
- 1 cup corn kernels (fresh or frozen)
- 1 small red onion, finely chopped
- 3 cloves garlic, minced
- 1 teaspoon cumin
- 1 teaspoon smoked paprika
- 1/2 teaspoon turmeric powder
- Salt and pepper to taste
- 1 cup tomato sauce
- 1/2 cup nutritional yeast
- Fresh cilantro for garnish

Instructions:

1. Preheat the oven to 375°F (190°C). Place halved bell peppers in a baking dish, cut side up.

2. In a pan over medium heat, sauté the finely chopped red onion and minced garlic until softened.

3. Add diced portobello mushrooms and chopped baby spinach to the pan. Sauté until the mushrooms release their moisture and the spinach wilts.

4. In a large bowl, combine cooked quinoa, black beans, corn, cumin, smoked paprika, turmeric powder, salt, and pepper. Add the sautéed mushroom and spinach mixture. Mix adequately.

5. Stuff each bell pepper half with the quinoa and vegetable mixture, pressing it down slightly.

6. In a small bowl, mix tomato sauce and nutritional yeast. Spoon the sauce over the stuffed peppers.

7. Cover the baking dish with foil and bake in the preheated oven for 25-30 minutes, or until the peppers are tender.

8. Garnish with fresh cilantro before serving.

Nutritional Information (per serving):

Carbs: 40g | **Fats:** 5g | **Fiber:** 10g | **Protein:** 12g

Harissa Spiced Chickpea Tagine

Prep Time: 20 minutes | **Cook Time:** 40 minutes | **Number of Servings:** 4

Ingredients:

- 2 cups dried chickpeas, soaked overnight and cooked
- 2 tablespoons olive oil
- 1 large onion, finely chopped
- 3 cloves garlic, minced
- 1 large carrot, diced
- 1 zucchini, diced
- 1 bell pepper, diced
- 1 can (14 oz) diced tomatoes
- 1/4 cup tomato paste
- 2 tablespoons harissa paste
- 1 teaspoon ground cumin
- 1 teaspoon ground coriander
- 1/2 teaspoon ground cinnamon
- 1/2 teaspoon ground turmeric
- 1/4 teaspoon cayenne pepper (adjust to taste)
- Salt and pepper to taste
- 2 cups vegetable broth
- 1 cup dried apricots, chopped
- Fresh cilantro for garnish
- Cooked couscous or quinoa for serving

Instructions:

1. Soak chickpeas overnight, then cook until tender. Set aside.

2. In a large tagine or pot, heat olive oil over medium heat. Add finely chopped onion and minced garlic. Sauté until the onion is translucent.

3. Add diced carrot, diced zucchini, and diced bell pepper to the tagine. Cook for 5-7 minutes until the vegetables start to soften.

4. Stir in diced tomatoes, tomato paste, and harissa paste. Mix adequately to combine.

5. Add ground cumin, ground coriander, ground cinnamon, ground turmeric, cayenne pepper, salt, and pepper. Stir the spices into the vegetable mixture.

6. Pour vegetable broth into the tagine, stirring to combine. Bring the mixture to a simmer.

7. Add cooked chickpeas and chopped dried apricots to the tagine. Stir adequately and let it simmer for an additional 20-25 minutes.

8. Taste and adjust the seasoning if needed. If the tagine gets too dry, add more vegetable broth.

9. Serve the Harissa Spiced Chickpea Tagine over cooked couscous or quinoa. Garnish with fresh cilantro.

Nutritional Information (per serving):

Carbs: 55g | **Fats:** 8g | **Fiber:** 12g | **Protein:** 14g

Coconut Quinoa Pilaf with Roasted Vegetables

Prep Time: 20 minutes | **Cook Time:** 25 minutes | **Number of Servings:** 4

Ingredients:

- 1 cup quinoa, rinsed
- 1 can (400ml) coconut milk
- 2 cups broccoli florets
- 1 large carrot, sliced into rounds
- 1 red bell pepper, diced
- 1 yellow bell pepper, diced
- 1 zucchini, sliced
- 1 red onion, thinly sliced
- 3 cloves garlic, minced
- 2 tablespoons coconut oil
- 1 teaspoon ground turmeric
- 1 teaspoon ground cumin
- 1/2 teaspoon ground coriander
- Salt and pepper to taste
- Fresh cilantro for garnish

Instructions:

1. Preheat the oven to 400°F (200°C).

2. In a saucepan, combine quinoa and coconut milk. Bring to a boil, then reduce heat to low, cover, and simmer for 15 minutes or until the quinoa is cooked and liquid is absorbed.

3. On a baking sheet, toss broccoli florets, carrot rounds, diced red bell pepper, diced yellow bell pepper, sliced zucchini, thinly sliced red onion, and minced garlic with coconut oil. Sprinkle ground turmeric, ground cumin, ground coriander, salt, and pepper. Toss to coat evenly.

4. Roast the seasoned vegetables in the preheated oven for 20-25 minutes, or until they are tender and slightly caramelized.

5. Once the quinoa is cooked, fluff it with a fork to separate the grains.

6. In a large bowl, put together the cooked quinoa with the roasted vegetables. Mix adequately to incorporate the flavors.

7. Taste and adjust the seasoning if necessary. Add more salt and pepper as needed.

8. Garnish the Coconut Quinoa Pilaf with fresh cilantro before serving.

Nutritional Information (per serving):

- **Carbs:** 40g
- **Fats:** 18g
- **Fiber:** 8g
- **Protein:** 10g

Lentil Walnut Burger with Avocado Aioli

Prep Time: 20 minutes | **Cook Time:** 15 minutes | **Number of Servings:** 4

Ingredients:

For Lentil Walnut Burger:

- 1 cup dried green lentils, cooked
- 1 cup walnuts, finely chopped
- 1 cup oats, ground into flour
- 1 flax egg (1 tablespoon ground flaxseed mixed with 3 tablespoons water)
- 1 small red onion, finely diced
- 2 cloves garlic, minced
- 1 teaspoon ground cumin
- 1 teaspoon smoked paprika
- 1/2 teaspoon ground coriander
- Salt and pepper to taste
- 2 tablespoons olive oil (for cooking)

For Avocado Aioli:

- 1 ripe avocado, mashed
- 1 clove garlic, minced
- 2 tablespoons vegan mayonnaise
- 1 tablespoon lemon juice
- Salt and pepper to taste

For Serving:

- Whole-grain burger buns
- Lettuce leaves
- Tomato slices
- Red onion rings

Instructions:

1. Cook dried green lentils according to package instructions. Drain and set aside.
2. In a small bowl, mix ground flaxseed with water to create a flax egg. Let it sit for 5 minutes until it thickens.
3. In a large bowl, combine cooked lentils, finely chopped walnuts, oat flour, flax egg, finely diced red onion, minced garlic, ground cumin, smoked paprika, ground coriander, salt, and pepper. Mix until well combined.
4. Divide the mixture into 4 equal portions and shape them into burger patties.
5. Heat olive oil in a pan over medium heat. Cook the lentil walnut patties for about 6-8 minutes per side, or until they are golden brown and cooked through.
6. In a bowl, mash the ripe avocado. Add minced garlic, vegan mayonnaise, lemon juice, salt, and pepper. Mix adequately to create the avocado aioli.
7. Toast whole-grain burger buns. Spread a generous amount of avocado aioli on the buns. Place the cooked lentil walnut patties on the buns and top with lettuce leaves, tomato slices, and red onion rings.
8. Serve the Lentil Walnut Burger with Avocado Aioli immediately.

Nutritional Information (per serving):

Carbs: 45g | **Fats:** 22g | **Fiber:** 12g | **Protein:** 15g

Moroccan Spiced Eggplant and Couscous Skillet

Prep Time: 20 minutes | **Cook Time:** 25 minutes | **Number of Servings:** 4

Ingredients:

- 1 cup couscous
- 2 cups vegetable broth
- 2 medium eggplants, diced
- 1 large onion, finely chopped
- 3 cloves garlic, minced
- 1 can (14 oz) chickpeas, drained and rinsed
- 1 can (14 oz) diced tomatoes
- 1/2 cup dried apricots, chopped
- 1/4 cup sliced almonds
- 2 tablespoons olive oil
- 1 teaspoon ground cumin
- 1 teaspoon ground coriander
- 1 teaspoon ground cinnamon
- 1/2 teaspoon smoked paprika
- Salt and pepper to taste
- Fresh parsley for garnish

Instructions:

1. In a saucepan, bring vegetable broth to a boil. Add couscous, remove from heat, cover, and let it sit for 5 minutes. Fluff with a fork.

2. In a large skillet, heat olive oil over medium heat. Add finely chopped onion and minced garlic. Sauté until the onion is translucent.

3. Add diced eggplant to the skillet. Cook for 8-10 minutes, or until the eggplant is tender.

4. Sprinkle ground cumin, ground coriander, ground cinnamon, smoked paprika, salt, and pepper over the eggplant mixture. Stir to coat the eggplant in the spices.

5. Add drained and rinsed chickpeas, diced tomatoes (with their juices), and chopped dried apricots to the skillet. Stir adequately to combine.

6. Let the mixture simmer for 10-15 minutes, allowing the flavors to meld and the sauce to thicken.

7. Fluff the couscous with a fork and spread it on a serving platter, creating a bed for the Moroccan spiced eggplant mixture.

8. **Serve:** Spoon the spiced eggplant mixture over the couscous bed. Garnish with sliced almonds and fresh parsley.

Nutritional Information (per serving):

- **Carbs:** 60g
- **Fats:** 10g
- **Fiber:** 15g
- **Protein:** 12g

Walnut and Herb Crusted Tempeh Steaks

Prep Time: 15 minutes | **Cook Time:** 20 minutes | **Number of Servings:** 4

Ingredients:

- 2 packages (16 oz) tempeh
- 1 cup walnuts, finely chopped
- 1/2 cup fresh parsley, finely chopped
- 2 tablespoons nutritional yeast
- 1 tablespoon Dijon mustard
- 1 tablespoon lemon juice
- 2 cloves garlic, minced
- 1 teaspoon dried thyme
- 1 teaspoon dried rosemary
- Salt and pepper to taste
- 2 tablespoons olive oil (for cooking)

Instructions:

1. Preheat the oven to 375°F (190°C).

2. Cut each tempeh block into two equal-sized steaks. Steam the tempeh for 10 minutes to reduce bitterness.

3. In a bowl, combine finely chopped walnuts, finely chopped fresh parsley, nutritional yeast, Dijon mustard, lemon juice, minced garlic, dried thyme, dried rosemary, salt, and pepper. Mix adequately to form a cohesive crust.

4. Press each tempeh steak into the walnut and herb crust mixture, ensuring both sides are evenly coated.

5. In an oven-safe skillet, heat olive oil over medium heat. Sear the coated tempeh steaks for 2-3 minutes on each side until golden brown.

6. Transfer the skillet to the preheated oven and bake for an additional 12-15 minutes, or until the tempeh steaks are heated through and have a crispy crust.

7. Remove from the oven and let the tempeh steaks rest for a few minutes before serving.

8. **Optional:** Serve with your favorite side dishes or a light salad.

Nutritional Information (per serving):

- **Carbs:** 12g
- **Fats:** 20g
- **Fiber:** 6g
- **Protein:** 22g

Creamy Turmeric Polenta with Roasted Vegetables

Prep Time: 15 minutes | **Cook Time:** 30 minutes | **Number of Servings:** 4

Ingredients:

For Creamy Turmeric Polenta:

- 1 cup polenta
- 4 cups vegetable broth
- 1 can (14 oz) coconut milk
- 1 teaspoon ground turmeric
- Salt and pepper to taste
- 2 tablespoons nutritional yeast (optional)
- 2 tablespoons vegan butter

For Roasted Vegetables:

- 1 large sweet potato, peeled and diced
- 2 carrots, sliced into rounds
- 1 red bell pepper, diced
- 1 zucchini, sliced
- 1 red onion, sliced into wedges
- 3 tablespoons olive oil
- 1 teaspoon ground cumin
- 1 teaspoon smoked paprika
- Salt and pepper to taste

For Garnish:

- Fresh parsley, chopped
- Vegan feta cheese, crumbled (optional)

Instructions:

1. Preheat the oven to 400°F (200°C).

2. In a pot, bring vegetable broth and coconut milk to a boil. Gradually whisk in polenta, ensuring there are no lumps. Reduce heat to low, add ground turmeric, salt, and pepper. Cook, stirring frequently, until the polenta is creamy and fully cooked. Add nutritional yeast and vegan butter, mix adequately.

3. On a baking sheet, toss diced sweet potato, sliced carrots, diced red bell pepper, sliced zucchini, and sliced red onion with olive oil, ground cumin, smoked paprika, salt, and pepper. Roast in the preheated oven for 20-25 minutes or until the vegetables are tender and slightly caramelized.

4. Spoon the creamy turmeric polenta onto plates or a serving platter. Top with the roasted vegetables.

5. Garnish with chopped fresh parsley and crumbled vegan feta cheese if desired.

6. **Optional:** Drizzle with extra olive oil before serving.

Nutritional Information (per serving):

Carbs: 45g | **Fats:** 20g | **Fiber:** 8g | **Protein:** 6g

Moroccan Spiced Lentil and Eggplant Casserole

Prep Time: 25 minutes | **Cook Time:** 40 minutes | **Number of Servings:** 6

Ingredients:

- 1 cup brown lentils, uncooked
- 2 large eggplants, diced
- 1 large onion, finely chopped
- 3 cloves garlic, minced
- 1 can (14 oz) diced tomatoes
- 1 can (14 oz) chickpeas, drained and rinsed
- 1 cup vegetable broth
- 1/2 cup dried apricots, chopped
- 1/4 cup tomato paste
- 2 tablespoons olive oil
- 1 tablespoon ground cumin
- 1 tablespoon ground coriander
- 1 teaspoon ground cinnamon
- 1/2 teaspoon ground turmeric
- 1/4 teaspoon cayenne pepper (adjust to taste)
- Salt and pepper to taste
- Fresh cilantro for garnish

Instructions:

1. Cook brown lentils according to package instructions. Set aside.

2. Sprinkle diced eggplant with salt and let it sit for 15 minutes. Rinse and pat dry.

3. In a large oven-safe casserole dish, sauté finely chopped onion and minced garlic in olive oil until softened.

4. Add ground cumin, ground coriander, ground cinnamon, ground turmeric, cayenne pepper, salt, and pepper to the sautéed onion and garlic. Stir to coat.

5. Add the diced, dried eggplant to the casserole dish. Cook for 5-7 minutes until the eggplant starts to brown.

6. Stir in cooked brown lentils, diced tomatoes, chickpeas, vegetable broth, chopped dried apricots, and tomato paste. Mix adequately to combine all ingredients.

7. Cover the casserole dish and bake in a preheated oven at 375°F (190°C) for 25-30 minutes, or until the eggplant is tender.

8. Garnish the Moroccan Spiced Lentil and Eggplant Casserole with fresh cilantro before serving.

Nutritional Information (per serving):

- **Carbs:** 45g
- **Fats:** 8g
- **Fiber:** 12g
- **Protein:** 12g

Smoky Turmeric Grilled Portobello Mushrooms

Prep Time: 15 minutes | **Cook Time:** 10 minutes | **Number of Servings:** 4

Ingredients:

- 4 large portobello mushrooms, cleaned and stems removed
- 2 tablespoons olive oil
- 2 tablespoons tamari (gluten-free soy sauce)
- 1 teaspoon ground turmeric
- 1 teaspoon smoked paprika
- 1 teaspoon garlic powder
- 1/2 teaspoon liquid smoke
- 1/4 teaspoon black pepper
- Fresh parsley for garnish (optional)

Instructions:

1. Clean the portobello mushrooms and take out the stems.

2. In a bowl, whisk together olive oil, tamari, ground turmeric, smoked paprika, garlic powder, liquid smoke, and black pepper to create the marinade.

3. Place the portobello mushrooms in a shallow dish, gill side up. Pour the marinade over the mushrooms, ensuring they are well-coated. Let them marinate for at least 10 minutes.

4. Preheat the grill or grill pan over medium-high heat.

5. Place the marinated portobello mushrooms on the preheated grill, gill side down. Grill for 5 minutes on each side, or until the mushrooms are tender and have grill marks.

6. While grilling, baste the mushrooms with the remaining marinade to enhance the flavor.

7. Take out the grilled portobello mushrooms from the grill. Garnish with fresh parsley if desired. Serve them as a side dish, on a salad, or in a sandwich.

Nutritional Information (per serving):

- **Carbs:** 8g
- **Fats:** 6g
- **Fiber:** 3g
- **Protein:** 5g

Spaghetti Squash with Spinach and Pine Nut Pesto

Prep Time: 15 minutes | **Cook Time:** 40 minutes | **Number of Servings:** 4

Ingredients:

For Spaghetti Squash:

- 2 medium spaghetti squash
- 2 tablespoons olive oil
- Salt and pepper to taste

For Spinach and Pine Nut Pesto:

- 4 cups fresh spinach leaves
- 1/2 cup pine nuts
- 2 cloves garlic, minced
- 1/4 cup nutritional yeast
- 1/4 cup olive oil
- 1 tablespoon lemon juice
- Salt and pepper to taste

For Garnish:

- Fresh basil leaves
- Cherry tomatoes, halved (optional)
- Vegan Parmesan cheese (optional)

Instructions:

1. Preheat the oven to 400°F (200°C).

2. Cut the spaghetti squash in half lengthwise. Scoop out the seeds. Brush the cut sides with olive oil and sprinkle with salt and pepper. Place them on a baking sheet, cut side down. Roast in the preheated oven for 35-40 minutes, or until the squash is tender.

3. In a food processor, combine fresh spinach, pine nuts, minced garlic, nutritional yeast, olive oil, lemon juice, salt, and pepper. Blend until you achieve a smooth pesto consistency.

4. Once the spaghetti squash is cooked, use a fork to scrape the flesh into spaghetti-like strands.

5. In a large bowl, toss the spaghetti squash strands with the prepared spinach and pine nut pesto until well coated.

6. Divide the Spaghetti Squash with Spinach and Pine Nut Pesto among plates.

7. Garnish with fresh basil leaves and, if desired, halved cherry tomatoes and vegan Parmesan cheese.

Nutritional Information (per serving):

Carbs: 20g | **Fats:** 18g | **Fiber:** 5g | **Protein:** 5g

Quinoa and Black Bean Stuffed Bell Peppers

Prep Time: 20 minutes | **Cook Time:** 30 minutes | **Number of Servings:** 6

Ingredients:

- 1 cup quinoa, cooked
- 6 large bell peppers, halved and seeds removed
- 1 can (15 oz) black beans, drained and rinsed
- 1 cup corn kernels (fresh or frozen)
- 1 cup cherry tomatoes, diced
- 1 red onion, finely chopped
- 2 cloves garlic, minced
- 1 teaspoon ground cumin
- 1 teaspoon smoked paprika
- 1/2 teaspoon chili powder
- Salt and pepper to taste
- 1 cup tomato sauce
- 1 cup vegan cheese, shredded (optional)
- Fresh cilantro for garnish

Instructions:

1. Preheat the oven to 375°F (190°C).
2. Cut the bell peppers in half, removing seeds and membranes. Place them in a baking dish, cut side up.
3. Cook quinoa according to package instructions. Set aside.
4. In a large bowl, combine cooked quinoa, black beans, corn kernels, diced cherry tomatoes, finely chopped red onion, minced garlic, ground cumin, smoked paprika, chili powder, salt, and pepper. Mix adequately.
5. Spoon the quinoa and black bean mixture into each bell pepper half, pressing down gently.
6. Pour tomato sauce over the stuffed bell peppers.
7. Cover the baking dish with aluminum foil and bake in the preheated oven for 25-30 minutes, or until the peppers are tender.
8. If desired, sprinkle shredded vegan cheese over the stuffed peppers during the last 5 minutes of baking until melted.
9. Garnish with fresh cilantro and serve the Quinoa and Black Bean Stuffed Bell Peppers.

Nutritional Information (per serving):

- **Carbs:** 45g
- **Fats:** 5g
- **Fiber:** 10g
- **Protein:** 10g

Chapter 6: Sides

Garlic Roasted Brussels Sprouts

Prep Time: 15 minutes | **Cook Time:** 25 minutes | **Servings:** 4

Ingredients:

- 1 pound Brussels sprouts, trimmed and halved
- 3 tablespoons olive oil
- 4 cloves garlic, minced
- 1 teaspoon smoked paprika
- 1/2 teaspoon sea salt
- 1/4 teaspoon black pepper

Instructions:

1. Preheat your oven to 400°F (200°C).
2. In a large bowl, toss the halved Brussels sprouts with olive oil, minced garlic, smoked paprika, sea salt, and black pepper until evenly coated.
3. Spread the Brussels sprouts in a single layer on a baking sheet.
4. Roast in the preheated oven for 25 minutes or until the sprouts are golden brown and crispy on the edges, tossing halfway through for even cooking.
5. Remove from the oven and serve immediately.

Nutritional Information (per serving):

- **Carbs:** 12g
- **Fats:** 9g
- **Fiber:** 4g
- **Protein:** 3g

Turmeric Cauliflower Mash

Prep Time: 10 minutes | **Cook Time:** 20 minutes | **Servings:** 4

Ingredients:

- 1 large head cauliflower, chopped into florets
- 2 tablespoons olive oil
- 3 cloves garlic, minced
- 1 teaspoon ground turmeric
- 1/2 teaspoon ground cumin
- 1/2 teaspoon sea salt
- 1/4 teaspoon black pepper
- 1/2 cup unsweetened almond milk
- Fresh parsley, chopped (for garnish)

Instructions:

1. Steam the cauliflower florets until fork-tender, about 10-12 minutes.
2. While the cauliflower is steaming, heat olive oil in a pan over medium heat. Add minced garlic and sauté until fragrant.
3. Add ground turmeric, ground cumin, sea salt, and black pepper to the sautéed garlic. Stir to combine and cook for an additional 1-2 minutes.
4. Once the cauliflower is cooked, transfer it to a large bowl. Add the spice mixture and almond milk.
5. Use a potato masher or immersion blender to mash the cauliflower until smooth and creamy.
6. Adjust seasoning if needed and garnish with fresh chopped parsley before serving.

Nutritional Information (per serving):

- **Carbs:** 8g
- **Fats:** 7g
- **Fiber:** 4g
- **Protein:** 3g

Ginger Glazed Carrot Ribbons

Prep Time: 15 minutes | **Cook Time:** 10 minutes | **Servings:** 4

Ingredients:

- 8 large carrots, peeled and thinly ribboned
- 2 tablespoons coconut oil
- 2 tablespoons fresh ginger, grated
- 2 tablespoons maple syrup
- 1 tablespoon tamari (gluten-free soy sauce)
- 1/2 teaspoon ground turmeric
- 1/4 teaspoon black pepper
- Sesame seeds (for garnish)
- Fresh cilantro, chopped (for garnish)

Instructions:

1. Peel the carrots and, using a vegetable peeler, create thin ribbons by running the peeler along the length of each carrot.

2. In a large pan, heat coconut oil over medium heat. Add the grated ginger and sauté for 1-2 minutes until fragrant.

3. Add the carrot ribbons to the pan, tossing to coat them in the ginger-infused oil.

4. In a small bowl, mix together maple syrup, tamari, ground turmeric, and black pepper. Pour the mixture over the carrot ribbons.

5. Cook the carrot ribbons for 5-7 minutes, stirring frequently, until they are tender yet still have a slight crunch.

6. Garnish with sesame seeds and freshly chopped cilantro before serving.

Nutritional Information (per serving):

- **Carbs:** 18g
- **Fats:** 7g
- **Fiber:** 4g
- **Protein:** 2g

Lemon Herb Quinoa Pilaf

Prep Time: 15 minutes | **Cook Time:** 20 minutes | **Servings:** 4

Ingredients:

- 1 cup quinoa, rinsed and drained
- 2 cups vegetable broth
- 1 tablespoon olive oil
- 1 onion, finely diced
- 2 cloves garlic, minced
- 1 teaspoon dried thyme
- 1 teaspoon dried rosemary
- Zest of 1 lemon
- Juice of 1 lemon
- 1/4 cup fresh parsley, chopped
- Salt and pepper to taste

Instructions:

1. In a medium saucepan, bring vegetable broth to a boil. Add quinoa, reduce heat to low, cover, and simmer for 15 minutes or until the quinoa is cooked and the liquid is absorbed.

2. While the quinoa is cooking, heat olive oil in a large pan over medium heat. Add finely diced onions and sauté until translucent.

3. Add minced garlic to the onions and sauté for an additional 1-2 minutes until fragrant.

4. Stir in dried thyme and dried rosemary to the onion and garlic mixture.

5. Once the quinoa is cooked, fluff it with a fork and add it to the pan with the onion and herb mixture.

6. Add lemon zest, lemon juice, and chopped fresh parsley to the quinoa mixture. Toss gently to combine.

7. Season with salt and pepper to taste.

8. Serve the Lemon Herb Quinoa Pilaf warm.

Nutritional Information (per serving):

- **Carbs:** 37g
- **Fats:** 6g
- **Fiber:** 5g
- **Protein:** 8g

Baked Sweet Potato Slices with Rosemary

Prep Time: 15 minutes | **Cook Time:** 25 minutes | **Servings:** 4

Ingredients:

- 2 large sweet potatoes, peeled and sliced into 1/4-inch rounds
- 2 tablespoons olive oil
- 1 tablespoon fresh rosemary, finely chopped
- 1/2 teaspoon garlic powder
- 1/2 teaspoon onion powder
- 1/2 teaspoon smoked paprika
- Sea salt and black pepper to taste

Instructions:

1. Preheat the oven to 425°F (220°C).
2. In a large bowl, toss the sweet potato rounds with olive oil, finely chopped fresh rosemary, garlic powder, onion powder, smoked paprika, sea salt, and black pepper until well coated.
3. Arrange the sweet potato slices in a single layer on a baking sheet lined with parchment paper.
4. Bake in the preheated oven for 25 minutes or until the sweet potatoes are tender and golden brown, flipping halfway through for even cooking.
5. Remove from the oven and let them rest for a few minutes before serving.

Nutritional Information (per serving):

- **Carbs:** 26g
- **Fats:** 7g
- **Fiber:** 4g
- **Protein:** 2g

Green Bean Almondine with Lemon

Prep Time: 15 minutes | **Cook Time:** 10 minutes | **Servings:** 4

Ingredients:

- 1 pound fresh green beans, ends trimmed
- 2 tablespoons olive oil
- 1/2 cup almonds, sliced
- 2 cloves garlic, thinly sliced
- Zest of 1 lemon
- Juice of 1 lemon
- Salt and pepper to taste
- Fresh parsley, chopped (for garnish)

Instructions:

1. Bring a large pot of salted water to a boil. Add the trimmed green beans and blanch for 3-4 minutes until they are bright green and slightly tender. Drain and immediately transfer to a bowl of ice water to stop the cooking process. Drain again and set aside.

2. In a large pan, heat olive oil over medium heat. Add sliced almonds and sauté until they are golden brown and fragrant.

3. Add thinly sliced garlic to the pan with almonds and sauté for an additional 1-2 minutes until the garlic is softened but not browned.

4. Add the blanched green beans to the pan, tossing them with the almond and garlic mixture.

5. Drizzle lemon juice over the green beans and sprinkle lemon zest on top. Toss to combine and cook for an additional 2-3 minutes until the beans are heated through.

6. Season with salt and pepper to taste.

7. Garnish with chopped fresh parsley before serving.

Nutritional Information (per serving):

- **Carbs:** 12g
- **Fats:** 10g
- **Fiber:** 5g
- **Protein:** 4g

<u>Miso Glazed Eggplant Slices</u>

Prep Time: 20 minutes | **Cook Time:** 15 minutes | **Servings:** 4

Ingredients:

- 2 large eggplants, sliced into 1/2-inch rounds
- 3 tablespoons white miso paste
- 2 tablespoons maple syrup
- 2 tablespoons rice vinegar
- 1 tablespoon sesame oil
- 1 tablespoon tamari (gluten-free soy sauce)
- 2 cloves garlic, minced
- 1 tablespoon fresh ginger, grated
- Sesame seeds and green onions, sliced (for garnish)

Instructions:

1. Preheat the oven to 400°F (200°C).
2. Lay the eggplant slices on a baking sheet lined with parchment paper.
3. In a small bowl, whisk together white miso paste, maple syrup, rice vinegar, sesame oil, tamari, minced garlic, and grated fresh ginger.
4. Brush the miso glaze generously over each eggplant slice, ensuring they are well coated on both sides.
5. Bake in the preheated oven for 15 minutes or until the eggplant is tender and the edges are caramelized, flipping halfway through for even glazing.
6. Remove from the oven and sprinkle sesame seeds and sliced green onions on top before serving.

Nutritional Information (per serving):

- **Carbs:** 20g
- **Fats:** 6g
- **Fiber:** 9g
- **Protein:** 3g

Turmeric Dill Pickled Cucumbers

Prep Time: 15 minutes | **Cook Time:** 0 minutes (no cooking required) | **Servings:** 4

Ingredients:

- 4 medium cucumbers, thinly sliced
- 1 cup white vinegar
- 1 cup water
- 2 tablespoons maple syrup
- 1 tablespoon sea salt
- 1 teaspoon ground turmeric
- 1 teaspoon mustard seeds
- 1 teaspoon whole black peppercorns
- 4 cloves garlic, sliced
- 4 sprigs fresh dill

Instructions:

1. In a medium saucepan, combine white vinegar, water, maple syrup, sea salt, ground turmeric, mustard seeds, and whole black peppercorns. Bring the mixture to a gentle boil over medium heat, stirring until the salt and maple syrup are dissolved. Remove from heat and let it cool to room temperature.

2. While the brine is cooling, layer the thinly sliced cucumbers, sliced garlic, and fresh dill sprigs in a clean, sterilized jar.

3. Once the brine has cooled, pour it over the cucumbers in the jar, ensuring they are completely submerged in the liquid.

4. Seal the jar tightly and refrigerate for at least 24 hours before serving to allow the flavors to develop.

Nutritional Information (per serving):

- **Carbs:** 10g
- **Fats:** 0g
- **Fiber:** 2g
- **Protein:** 1g

Roasted Garlic and Herb Quinoa

Prep Time: 15 minutes | **Cook Time:** 20 minutes | **Servings:** 4

Ingredients:

- 1 cup quinoa, rinsed and drained
- 2 cups vegetable broth
- 1 head garlic
- 2 tablespoons olive oil
- 1 teaspoon dried thyme
- 1 teaspoon dried rosemary
- 1 teaspoon dried oregano
- Salt and black pepper to taste
- Fresh parsley, chopped (for garnish)

Instructions:

1. Preheat the oven to 400°F (200°C).

2. Cut the top off the head of garlic to expose the cloves. Place the garlic head on a piece of foil, drizzle with a little olive oil, and wrap it tightly. Roast in the preheated oven for about 30 minutes or until the cloves are soft and golden. Allow it to cool before squeezing the roasted garlic out of the cloves.

3. In a medium saucepan, bring vegetable broth to a boil. Add quinoa, reduce heat to low, cover, and simmer for 15 minutes or until the quinoa is cooked and the liquid is absorbed.

4. While the quinoa is cooking, heat 2 tablespoons of olive oil in a pan over medium heat. Add the squeezed roasted garlic, dried thyme, dried rosemary, and dried oregano. Cook for 2-3 minutes until the herbs are fragrant.

5. Once the quinoa is cooked, fluff it with a fork and add it to the pan with the roasted garlic and herb mixture.

6. Toss the quinoa until it is well-coated with the garlic and herbs. Season with salt and black pepper to taste.

7. Garnish with chopped fresh parsley before serving.

Nutritional Information (per serving):

- **Carbs:** 35g
- **Fats:** 9g
- **Fiber:** 5g
- **Protein:** 7g

Lemon Thyme Roasted Sweet Potatoes

Prep Time: 15 minutes | **Cook Time:** 25 minutes | **Servings:** 4

Ingredients:

- 4 medium sweet potatoes, peeled and cut into 1-inch cubes
- 3 tablespoons olive oil
- Zest of 1 lemon
- Juice of 1 lemon
- 2 tablespoons fresh thyme leaves
- 1 teaspoon garlic powder
- Salt and black pepper to taste

Instructions:

1. Preheat the oven to 425°F (220°C).
2. In a large bowl, toss the sweet potato cubes with olive oil, lemon zest, lemon juice, fresh thyme leaves, garlic powder, salt, and black pepper until well coated.
3. Spread the sweet potatoes in a single layer on a baking sheet lined with parchment paper.
4. Roast in the preheated oven for 25 minutes or until the sweet potatoes are tender and golden brown, tossing halfway through for even roasting.
5. Remove from the oven and transfer the roasted sweet potatoes to a serving dish.
6. Garnish with additional fresh thyme leaves before serving.

Nutritional Information (per serving):

- **Carbs:** 30g
- **Fats:** 9g
- **Fiber:** 5g
- **Protein:** 3g

Basil Pesto Zucchini Ribbons

Prep Time: 20 minutes | **Cook Time:** 0 minutes (no cooking required) | **Servings:** 4

Ingredients:

- 4 medium zucchinis
- 2 cups fresh basil leaves
- 1/2 cup raw walnuts
- 2 cloves garlic, minced
- 1/2 cup nutritional yeast
- 1/2 cup olive oil
- Juice of 1 lemon
- Salt and black pepper to taste
- Cherry tomatoes, halved (for garnish)

Instructions:

1. Using a vegetable peeler or a spiralizer, create thin ribbons or noodles with the zucchinis.
2. In a food processor, combine fresh basil leaves, raw walnuts, minced garlic, nutritional yeast, olive oil, and lemon juice. Process until the mixture forms a smooth pesto.
3. Season the pesto with salt and black pepper to taste, adjusting as needed.
4. In a large bowl, toss the zucchini ribbons with the basil pesto until well coated.
5. Serve the zucchini ribbons topped with halved cherry tomatoes.

Nutritional Information (per serving):

- **Carbs:** 10g
- **Fats:** 25g
- **Fiber:** 4g
- **Protein:** 5g

Almond and Cranberry Quinoa Stuffing

Prep Time: 15 minutes | **Cook Time:** 20 minutes | **Servings:** 6

Ingredients:

- 1 cup quinoa, rinsed and drained
- 2 cups vegetable broth
- 2 tablespoons olive oil
- 1 onion, finely diced
- 2 celery stalks, finely diced
- 1 cup sliced almonds
- 1/2 cup dried cranberries
- 1 teaspoon dried thyme
- 1 teaspoon dried rosemary
- 1 teaspoon dried sage
- Salt and black pepper to taste
- Fresh parsley, chopped (for garnish)

Instructions:

1. In a medium saucepan, bring vegetable broth to a boil. Add quinoa, reduce heat to low, cover, and simmer for 15 minutes or until the quinoa is cooked and the liquid is absorbed.

2. While the quinoa is cooking, heat olive oil in a large pan over medium heat. Add finely diced onions and celery. Sauté until the vegetables are softened.

3. Add sliced almonds to the pan and toast them until they are golden brown and fragrant.

4. Stir in dried cranberries, dried thyme, dried rosemary, and dried sage. Cook for an additional 2-3 minutes to allow the flavors to meld.

5. Once the quinoa is cooked, add it to the pan with the almond and cranberry mixture. Toss everything together until well combined.

6. Season with salt and black pepper to taste.

7. Garnish with chopped fresh parsley before serving.

Nutritional Information (per serving):

- **Carbs:** 30g
- **Fats:** 12g
- **Fiber:** 5g
- **Protein:** 7g

Turmeric Infused Couscous Pilaf

Prep Time: 10 minutes | **Cook Time:** 15 minutes | **Servings:** 4

Ingredients:

- 1 cup couscous
- 1 3/4 cups vegetable broth
- 2 tablespoons olive oil
- 1 onion, finely diced
- 2 carrots, finely diced
- 1 red bell pepper, finely diced
- 1 teaspoon ground turmeric
- 1/2 teaspoon ground cumin
- 1/2 teaspoon ground coriander
- Salt and black pepper to taste
- Fresh cilantro, chopped (for garnish)

Instructions:

1. In a medium saucepan, bring vegetable broth to a boil. Stir in couscous, cover, and remove from heat. Let it sit for 5 minutes until the couscous absorbs the liquid. Fluff with a fork.

2. While the couscous is resting, heat olive oil in a large pan over medium heat. Add finely diced onions, carrots, and red bell pepper. Sauté until the vegetables are softened.

3. Stir in ground turmeric, ground cumin, and ground coriander. Cook for an additional 2-3 minutes until the spices are fragrant.

4. Add the fluffed couscous to the pan with the sautéed vegetables and spices. Toss until well combined.

5. Season with salt and black pepper to taste.

6. Garnish with chopped fresh cilantro before serving.

Nutritional Information (per serving):

- **Carbs:** 40g
- **Fats:** 7g
- **Fiber:** 5g
- **Protein:** 5g

Garlic and Herb Roasted Brussels Sprouts

Prep Time: 15 minutes | **Cook Time:** 25 minutes | **Servings:** 4

Ingredients:

- 1 pound Brussels sprouts, trimmed and halved
- 3 tablespoons olive oil
- 4 cloves garlic, minced
- 1 teaspoon dried thyme
- 1 teaspoon dried rosemary
- 1/2 teaspoon sea salt
- 1/4 teaspoon black pepper

Instructions:

1. Preheat your oven to 400°F (200°C).
2. In a large bowl, toss the halved Brussels sprouts with olive oil, minced garlic, dried thyme, dried rosemary, sea salt, and black pepper until evenly coated.
3. Spread the Brussels sprouts in a single layer on a baking sheet.
4. Roast in the preheated oven for 25 minutes or until the sprouts are golden brown and crispy on the edges, tossing halfway through for even cooking.
5. Remove from the oven and serve immediately.

Nutritional Information (per serving):

- **Carbs:** 12g
- **Fats:** 9g
- **Fiber:** 4g
- **Protein:** 3g

Green Beans with Turmeric Almond Butter

Prep Time: 15 minutes | **Cook Time:** 10 minutes | **Servings:** 4

Ingredients:

- 1 pound green beans, ends trimmed
- 3 tablespoons almond butter
- 2 tablespoons olive oil
- 1 teaspoon ground turmeric
- 2 cloves garlic, minced
- 1 tablespoon maple syrup
- 1 tablespoon tamari (gluten-free soy sauce)
- 1/4 teaspoon black pepper
- Sliced almonds (for garnish)
- Fresh parsley, chopped (for garnish)

Instructions:

1. In a large pot of boiling water, blanch the green beans for 3-4 minutes until they are bright green and slightly tender. Drain and transfer to a bowl of ice water to stop the cooking process. Drain again and set aside.

2. In a small bowl, whisk together almond butter, olive oil, ground turmeric, minced garlic, maple syrup, tamari, and black pepper to create a smooth sauce.

3. Heat the almond butter sauce in a large pan over medium heat.

4. Add the blanched green beans to the pan, tossing to coat them in the turmeric almond butter sauce.

5. Cook for an additional 2-3 minutes until the green beans are heated through.

6. Garnish with sliced almonds and chopped fresh parsley before serving.

Nutritional Information (per serving):

- **Carbs:** 14g
- **Fats:** 14g
- **Fiber:** 5g
- **Protein:** 6g

Lemon Turmeric Roasted Fingerling Potatoes

Prep Time: 15 minutes | **Cook Time:** 30 minutes | **Servings:** 4

Ingredients:

- 1.5 pounds fingerling potatoes, halved lengthwise
- 3 tablespoons olive oil
- Zest of 1 lemon
- Juice of 1 lemon
- 1 teaspoon ground turmeric
- 1 teaspoon dried thyme
- 1/2 teaspoon garlic powder
- 1/2 teaspoon onion powder
- Sea salt and black pepper to taste
- Fresh parsley, chopped (for garnish)

Instructions:

1. Preheat your oven to 425°F (220°C).
2. In a large bowl, toss the halved fingerling potatoes with olive oil, lemon zest, lemon juice, ground turmeric, dried thyme, garlic powder, onion powder, sea salt, and black pepper until well coated.
3. Spread the potatoes in a single layer on a baking sheet.
4. Roast in the preheated oven for 30 minutes or until the potatoes are golden brown and crispy, tossing halfway through for even roasting.
5. Remove from the oven and transfer the roasted fingerling potatoes to a serving dish.
6. Garnish with chopped fresh parsley before serving.

Nutritional Information (per serving):

- **Carbs:** 32g
- **Fats:** 9g
- **Fiber:** 4g
- **Protein:** 3g

Coconut Cilantro Lime Rice

Prep Time: 10 minutes | **Cook Time:** 20 minutes | **Servings:** 4

Ingredients:

- 1 cup white rice
- 1 cup coconut milk
- 1 cup water
- 1/2 cup shredded coconut
- 1/4 cup fresh cilantro, chopped
- Zest of 1 lime
- Juice of 1 lime
- Salt to taste

Instructions:

1. Rinse the white rice under cold water until the water runs clear.
2. In a saucepan, put together the rinsed rice, coconut milk, and water. Bring to a boil.
3. Reduce the heat to low, cover, and simmer for 15-20 minutes or until the rice is tender and has absorbed the liquid.
4. While the rice is cooking, toast the shredded coconut in a dry pan over medium heat until golden brown. Set aside.
5. Once the rice is cooked, fluff it with a fork and add chopped fresh cilantro, lime zest, and lime juice. Mix adequately.
6. Season with salt to taste.
7. Serve the Coconut Cilantro Lime Rice topped with toasted shredded coconut.

Nutritional Information (per serving):

- **Carbs:** 45g
- **Fats:** 17g
- **Fiber:** 2g
- **Protein:** 4g

Spiced Chickpea and Zucchini Fritters

Prep Time: 15 minutes | **Cook Time:** 15 minutes | **Servings:** 4

Ingredients:

- 1 can (15 oz) chickpeas, drained and rinsed
- 1 zucchini, grated
- 1/2 red onion, finely chopped
- 2 cloves garlic, minced
- 1/4 cup fresh parsley, chopped

- 1 teaspoon ground cumin
- 1 teaspoon ground coriander
- 1/2 teaspoon smoked paprika
- 3 tablespoons chickpea flour
- Salt and black pepper to taste
- 2 tablespoons olive oil (for cooking)

Instructions:

1. In a food processor, combine chickpeas, grated zucchini, chopped red onion, minced garlic, fresh parsley, ground cumin, ground coriander, smoked paprika, chickpea flour, salt, and black pepper. Pulse until the mixture is well combined but still has some texture.

2. Transfer the mixture to a bowl and let it rest for 5 minutes to allow the chickpea flour to absorb moisture.

3. Heat olive oil in a pan over medium heat.

4. Form the chickpea mixture into small patties and place them in the heated pan.

5. Cook for 3-4 minutes on each side or until the fritters are golden brown and cooked through.

6. Remove from the pan and place on a paper towel to absorb any excess oil.

7. Serve the Spiced Chickpea and Zucchini Fritters warm.

Nutritional Information (per serving):

- **Carbs:** 22g
- **Fats:** 9g
- **Fiber:** 6g
- **Protein:** 7g

Chapter 7: Smoothies and Beverages

Pineapple Turmeric Smoothie

Prep Time: 10 minutes | **Cook Time:** 0 minutes | **Servings:** 2

Ingredients:

- 2 cups fresh pineapple chunks
- 1 cup coconut milk
- 1 medium banana, peeled and sliced
- 1 teaspoon turmeric powder
- 1 tablespoon chia seeds
- 1 cup kale leaves, stems removed
- 1/2 cup cucumber, peeled and sliced
- 1 tablespoon fresh ginger, grated
- 1 tablespoon flaxseeds
- 1 cup ice cubes

Instructions:

1. In a blender, combine fresh pineapple chunks, coconut milk, banana, turmeric powder, chia seeds, kale leaves, cucumber, ginger, flaxseeds, and ice cubes.
2. Blend on high speed until the mixture reaches a smooth consistency.
3. Pour the smoothie into glasses and serve immediately.

Nutritional Information (per serving):

- Carbs: 38g
- Fats: 10g
- Fiber: 9g
- Protein: 5g

Berry Anti-Inflammatory Blast

Prep Time: 5 minutes | **Cook Time:** 0 minutes | **Servings:** 2

Ingredients:

- 1 cup blueberries
- 1 cup strawberries, hulled and halved
- 1/2 cup blackberries
- 1/2 cup raspberries
- 1 tablespoon ground flaxseeds
- 1 tablespoon hemp seeds
- 1 teaspoon turmeric powder
- 1 cup kale leaves, stems removed
- 1 medium banana, peeled and sliced
- 1 1/2 cups coconut water
- 1 cup ice cubes

Instructions:

1. In a blender, combine blueberries, strawberries, blackberries, raspberries, flaxseeds, hemp seeds, turmeric powder, kale leaves, banana, coconut water, and ice cubes.

2. Blend on high speed until the mixture reaches a smooth consistency.

3. Pour the anti-inflammatory berry blast into glasses and serve immediately.

Nutritional Information (per serving):

- Carbs: 40g
- Fats: 7g
- Fiber: 11g
- Protein: 4g

Mango Ginger Green Tea Infusion

Prep Time: 10 minutes | **Cook Time:** 5 minutes (steeping time) | **Servings:** 2

Ingredients:

- 2 cups hot water
- 2 green tea bags
- 1 cup fresh mango, peeled and diced
- 1 tablespoon fresh ginger, sliced
- 1 tablespoon agave syrup (or sweetener of choice)
- 1 tablespoon chia seeds
- 1 tablespoon mint leaves, chopped
- Ice cubes (optional)

Instructions:

1. In a teapot, pour hot water over the green tea bags and let them steep for 5 minutes.
2. Take out the tea bags and allow the green tea to cool to room temperature.
3. In a blender, combine fresh mango, sliced ginger, agave syrup, chia seeds, and mint leaves.
4. Pour the cooled green tea into the blender with the other ingredients.
5. Blend on high speed until the mixture is smooth and well combined.
6. Strain the mixture to remove any pulp, if desired.
7. Serve the mango ginger green tea infusion over ice cubes if you prefer a chilled drink.

Nutritional Information (per serving):

- Carbs: 24g
- Fats: 2g
- Fiber: 6g
- Protein: 2g

Golden Milk Smoothie

Prep Time: 10 minutes | **Cook Time:** 0 minutes | **Servings:** 2

Ingredients:

- 2 cups unsweetened almond milk
- 1 large banana, peeled and sliced
- 1/2 cup frozen pineapple chunks
- 1 teaspoon turmeric powder
- 1/2 teaspoon ground cinnamon
- 1/4 teaspoon ground ginger
- 1 tablespoon chia seeds
- 1 tablespoon almond butter
- 1 tablespoon maple syrup (or sweetener of choice)
- 1 cup ice cubes

Instructions:

1. In a blender, combine unsweetened almond milk, sliced banana, frozen pineapple chunks, turmeric powder, ground cinnamon, ground ginger, chia seeds, almond butter, and maple syrup.

2. Add ice cubes to the blender.

3. Blend on high speed until the golden milk smoothie reaches a creamy and smooth consistency.

4. Pour the smoothie into glasses and serve immediately.

Nutritional Information (per serving):

- Carbs: 35g
- Fats: 12g
- Fiber: 7g
- Protein: 5g

Cucumber Mint Cooler

Prep Time: 10 minutes | **Cook Time:** 0 minutes | **Servings:** 2

Ingredients:

- 2 cups cucumber, peeled and sliced

- 1/4 cup fresh mint leaves

- 1 tablespoon agave syrup (or sweetener of choice)

- 1 tablespoon fresh lime juice

- 2 cups coconut water

- 1 cup ice cubes

Instructions:

1. In a blender, combine peeled and sliced cucumber, fresh mint leaves, agave syrup, and fresh lime juice.

2. Add coconut water to the blender.

3. Blend on high speed until the cucumber and mint are fully incorporated.

4. Strain the mixture to remove any pulp, if desired.

5. Pour the cucumber mint cooler into glasses over ice cubes.

Nutritional Information (per serving):

- Carbs: 15g

- Fats: 0g

- Fiber: 2g

- Protein: 1g

Blueberry Basil Detox Elixir

Prep Time: 10 minutes | **Cook Time:** 0 minutes | **Servings:** 2

Ingredients:

- 1 cup blueberries
- 1/2 cup fresh basil leaves
- 1 tablespoon chia seeds
- 1 tablespoon lemon juice
- 1 tablespoon agave syrup (or sweetener of choice)
- 1/2 teaspoon spirulina powder
- 2 cups water
- Ice cubes (optional)

Instructions:

1. In a blender, combine blueberries, fresh basil leaves, chia seeds, lemon juice, agave syrup, and spirulina powder.
2. Add water to the blender.
3. Blend on high speed until the blueberry basil detox elixir is smooth and well combined.
4. Strain the mixture to remove any pulp, if desired.
5. Pour the elixir into glasses over ice cubes if you prefer a chilled drink.

Nutritional Information (per serving):

- Carbs: 22g
- Fats: 2g
- Fiber: 7g
- Protein: 3g

Kiwi Turmeric Immunity Smoothie

Prep Time: 10 minutes | **Cook Time:** 0 minutes | **Servings:** 2

Ingredients:

- 2 kiwis, peeled and sliced
- 1 cup pineapple chunks
- 1 teaspoon turmeric powder
- 1 tablespoon chia seeds
- 1 tablespoon flaxseeds
- 1 cup kale leaves, stems removed
- 1/2 avocado, peeled and diced
- 1 tablespoon agave syrup (or sweetener of choice)
- 1 1/2 cups almond milk
- 1 cup ice cubes

Instructions:

1. In a blender, combine peeled and sliced kiwis, pineapple chunks, turmeric powder, chia seeds, flaxseeds, kale leaves, diced avocado, agave syrup, almond milk, and ice cubes.

2. Blend on high speed until the kiwi turmeric immunity smoothie reaches a smooth consistency.

3. Pour the smoothie into glasses and serve immediately.

Nutritional Information (per serving):

- Carbs: 29g
- Fats: 11g
- Fiber: 10g
- Protein: 5g

Green Apple Ginger Detox Elixir

Prep Time: 10 minutes | **Cook Time:** 0 minutes | **Servings:** 2

Ingredients:

- 2 green apples, cored and sliced
- 1 tablespoon fresh ginger, sliced
- 1 tablespoon mint leaves
- 1 tablespoon chia seeds
- 1 tablespoon lemon juice
- 1 tablespoon agave syrup (or sweetener of choice)
- 2 cups water
- Ice cubes (optional)

Instructions:

1. In a blender, combine cored and sliced green apples, sliced fresh ginger, mint leaves, chia seeds, lemon juice, agave syrup, and water.

2. Blend on high speed until the green apple ginger detox elixir is smooth and well combined.

3. Strain the mixture to remove any pulp, if desired.

4. Pour the elixir into glasses over ice cubes if you prefer a chilled drink.

Nutritional Information (per serving):

- Carbs: 27g
- Fats: 1g
- Fiber: 8g
- Protein: 2g

Anti-Inflammatory Berry Beet Smoothie

Prep Time: 10 minutes | **Cook Time:** 0 minutes | **Servings:** 2

Ingredients:

- 1 cup mixed berries (blueberries, strawberries, blackberries, raspberries)
- 1 small beet, peeled and diced
- 1 cup spinach leaves
- 1 tablespoon chia seeds
- 1 tablespoon flaxseeds
- 1 tablespoon hemp seeds
- 1 tablespoon agave syrup (or sweetener of choice)
- 1 1/2 cups coconut water
- 1 cup ice cubes

Instructions:

1. In a blender, combine mixed berries, peeled and diced beet, spinach leaves, chia seeds, flaxseeds, hemp seeds, agave syrup, coconut water, and ice cubes.
2. Blend on high speed until the anti-inflammatory berry beet smoothie reaches a smooth consistency.
3. Pour the smoothie into glasses and serve immediately.

Nutritional Information (per serving):

- Carbs: 31g
- Fats: 8g
- Fiber: 10g
- Protein: 6g

Pineapple Mint Coconut Water Refresher

Prep Time: 10 minutes | **Cook Time:** 0 minutes | **Servings:** 2

Ingredients:

- 2 cups fresh pineapple chunks
- 1/4 cup fresh mint leaves
- 1 tablespoon chia seeds
- 1 tablespoon agave syrup (or sweetener of choice)
- 1 1/2 cups coconut water
- 1 cup ice cubes

Instructions:

1. In a blender, combine fresh pineapple chunks, fresh mint leaves, chia seeds, agave syrup, coconut water, and ice cubes.
2. Blend on high speed until the pineapple mint coconut water refresher is smooth and well combined.
3. Strain the mixture to remove any pulp, if desired.
4. Pour the refresher into glasses over ice cubes.

Nutritional Information (per serving):

- Carbs: 30g
- Fats: 1g
- Fiber: 6g
- Protein: 2g

Mango Turmeric Chia Seed Pudding Smoothie

Prep Time: 10 minutes (plus overnight for chia seed pudding) | **Cook Time:** 0 minutes | **Servings:** 2

Ingredients:

Chia Seed Pudding:

- 1/4 cup chia seeds
- 1 cup coconut milk
- 1 tablespoon agave syrup (or sweetener of choice)

Smoothie:

- 1 cup mango chunks
- 1 teaspoon turmeric powder
- 1 tablespoon flaxseeds
- 1 tablespoon almond butter
- 1 1/2 cups almond milk
- 1 cup ice cubes

Instructions:

Chia Seed Pudding (prepare the night before):

1. In a bowl, combine chia seeds, coconut milk, and agave syrup. Stir adequately.

2. Cover the bowl and refrigerate overnight or for at least 4 hours until the chia seeds absorb the liquid and form a pudding-like consistency.

Smoothie:

1. In a blender, combine mango chunks, turmeric powder, flaxseeds, almond butter, almond milk, and ice cubes.

2. Add the prepared chia seed pudding to the blender.

3. Blend on high speed until the mango turmeric chia seed pudding smoothie is smooth and well combined.

4. Pour the smoothie into glasses and serve immediately.

Nutritional Information (per serving):

- Carbs: 39g
- Fats: 18g
- Fiber: 11g
- Protein: 6g

<u>Spirulina Citrus Superfood Smoothie</u>

Prep Time: 10 minutes | **Cook Time:** 0 minutes | **Servings:** 2

Ingredients:

- 1 banana, peeled and sliced
- 1 orange, peeled and segmented
- 1/2 grapefruit, peeled and segmented
- 1 teaspoon spirulina powder
- 1 tablespoon chia seeds
- 1 tablespoon hemp seeds
- 1 tablespoon agave syrup (or sweetener of choice)
- 1 1/2 cups coconut water
- 1 cup ice cubes

Instructions:

1. In a blender, combine sliced banana, peeled and segmented orange, peeled and segmented grapefruit, spirulina powder, chia seeds, hemp seeds, agave syrup, coconut water, and ice cubes.

2. Blend on high speed until the spirulina citrus superfood smoothie reaches a smooth and vibrant consistency.

3. Pour the smoothie into glasses and serve immediately.

Nutritional Information (per serving):

- Carbs: 41g
- Fats: 6g
- Fiber: 9g
- Protein: 5g

Raspberry Turmeric Ginger Smoothie

Prep Time: 10 minutes | **Cook Time:** 0 minutes | **Servings:** 2

Ingredients:

- 1 cup raspberries
- 1 banana, peeled and sliced
- 1 teaspoon turmeric powder
- 1 tablespoon fresh ginger, sliced
- 1 tablespoon chia seeds
- 1 tablespoon flaxseeds
- 1 tablespoon agave syrup (or sweetener of choice)
- 1 1/2 cups almond milk
- 1 cup ice cubes

Instructions:

1. In a blender, combine raspberries, sliced banana, turmeric powder, sliced fresh ginger, chia seeds, flaxseeds, agave syrup, almond milk, and ice cubes.

2. Blend on high speed until the raspberry turmeric ginger smoothie reaches a smooth consistency.

3. Pour the smoothie into glasses and serve immediately.

Nutritional Information (per serving):

- Carbs: 37g
- Fats: 9g
- Fiber: 11g
- Protein: 4g

Detox Green Tea Infusion with Lemon and Mint

Prep Time: 5 minutes | **Cook Time:** 5 minutes (steeping time) | **Servings:** 2

Ingredients:

- 2 green tea bags
- 2 cups hot water
- 1 lemon, thinly sliced
- 10 fresh mint leaves
- 1 tablespoon agave syrup (or sweetener of choice)
- Ice cubes (optional)

Instructions:

1. Place green tea bags in a teapot, and pour hot water over them. Let them steep for 5 minutes.
2. Take out the tea bags, and add thinly sliced lemon and fresh mint leaves to the tea.
3. Allow the green tea infusion to cool to room temperature.
4. Stir in agave syrup to sweeten the infusion.
5. Strain the mixture to remove tea leaves and mint leaves, if desired.
6. Pour the detox green tea infusion into glasses over ice cubes, if preferred.

Nutritional Information (per serving):

- Carbs: 10g
- Fats: 0g
- Fiber: 2g
- Protein: 0g

Papaya Turmeric Immunity Elixir

Prep Time: 10 minutes | **Cook Time:** 0 minutes | **Servings:** 2

Ingredients:

- 2 cups fresh papaya chunks
- 1 teaspoon turmeric powder
- 1 tablespoon fresh ginger, sliced
- 1 tablespoon chia seeds
- 1 tablespoon agave syrup (or sweetener of choice)
- 1 1/2 cups coconut water
- 1 cup ice cubes

Instructions:

1. In a blender, combine fresh papaya chunks, turmeric powder, sliced fresh ginger, chia seeds, agave syrup, coconut water, and ice cubes.
2. Blend on high speed until the papaya turmeric immunity elixir is smooth and well combined.
3. Strain the mixture to remove any pulp, if desired.
4. Pour the elixir into glasses over ice cubes.

Nutritional Information (per serving):

- Carbs: 32g
- Fats: 3g
- Fiber: 7g
- Protein: 3g

Blueberry Lavender Almond Milk Smoothie

Prep Time: 10 minutes | **Cook Time:** 0 minutes | **Servings:** 2

Ingredients:

- 1 cup blueberries
- 1 teaspoon dried lavender flowers
- 1 banana, peeled and sliced
- 1 tablespoon almond butter
- 1 tablespoon chia seeds
- 1 tablespoon flaxseeds
- 2 cups almond milk
- 1 cup ice cubes

Instructions:

1. In a blender, combine blueberries, dried lavender flowers, sliced banana, almond butter, chia seeds, flaxseeds, almond milk, and ice cubes.

2. Blend on high speed until the blueberry lavender almond milk smoothie reaches a smooth consistency.

3. Pour the smoothie into glasses and serve immediately.

Nutritional Information (per serving):

- Carbs: 34g
- Fats: 11g
- Fiber: 10g
- Protein: 6g

Pineapple Basil Anti-Inflammatory Cooler

Prep Time: 10 minutes | **Cook Time:** 0 minutes | **Servings:** 2

Ingredients:

- 2 cups fresh pineapple chunks
- 1/4 cup fresh basil leaves
- 1 tablespoon chia seeds
- 1 tablespoon agave syrup (or sweetener of choice)
- 1 tablespoon lime juice
- 2 cups coconut water
- 1 cup ice cubes

Instructions:

1. In a blender, combine fresh pineapple chunks, fresh basil leaves, chia seeds, agave syrup, lime juice, coconut water, and ice cubes.

2. Blend on high speed until the pineapple basil anti-inflammatory cooler is smooth and well combined.

3. Strain the mixture to remove any pulp, if desired.

4. Pour the cooler into glasses over ice cubes.

Nutritional Information (per serving):

- Carbs: 31g
- Fats: 1g
- Fiber: 6g
- Protein: 2g

Orange Turmeric Mango Smoothie Bowl

Prep Time: 10 minutes | **Cook Time:** 0 minutes | **Servings:** 2

Ingredients:

Smoothie Bowl:

- 2 oranges, peeled and segmented
- 1 cup mango chunks
- 1 teaspoon turmeric powder
- 1 banana, peeled and sliced
- 1 tablespoon chia seeds
- 1 tablespoon flaxseeds
- 1 1/2 cups almond milk

Toppings:

- Sliced strawberries
- Fresh blueberries
- Granola
- Coconut flakes
- Fresh mint leaves

Instructions:

1. In a blender, combine peeled and segmented oranges, mango chunks, turmeric powder, sliced banana, chia seeds, flaxseeds, and almond milk.
2. Blend on high speed until the smoothie reaches a thick and creamy consistency.
3. Pour the smoothie into bowls.
4. Top the smoothie bowls with sliced strawberries, fresh blueberries, granola, coconut flakes, and fresh mint leaves.
5. Serve the orange turmeric mango smoothie bowls immediately.

Nutritional Information (per serving):

- Carbs: 55g
- Fats: 15g
- Fiber: 12g
- Protein: 7g

Chapter 8: Snacks and Appetizers

Turmeric Roasted Chickpeas

Prep Time: 10 minutes | **Cook Time:** 40 minutes | **Number of Servings:** 4

Ingredients:

- 2 cans (15 oz each) dried chickpeas, drained and rinsed
- 2 tablespoons olive oil
- 1 teaspoon ground turmeric
- 1 teaspoon ground cumin
- 1 teaspoon smoked paprika
- 1/2 teaspoon garlic powder
- 1/2 teaspoon onion powder
- 1/2 teaspoon sea salt
- 1/4 teaspoon black pepper

Instructions:

1. Preheat the oven to 400°F (200°C).

2. In a large bowl, put together the drained and rinsed chickpeas with olive oil, turmeric, cumin, smoked paprika, garlic powder, onion powder, sea salt, and black pepper. Mix adequately to ensure the chickpeas are evenly coated with the spices.

3. Spread the seasoned chickpeas in a single layer on a baking sheet lined with parchment paper.

4. Roast in the preheated oven for 35-40 minutes, or until the chickpeas are golden brown and crispy. Shake the pan or stir the chickpeas halfway through the cooking time for even roasting.

5. Remove from the oven and let the chickpeas cool for a few minutes before serving.

Nutritional Information (Per Serving):

- **Carbs:** 30g
- **Fats:** 10g
- **Fiber:** 7g
- **Protein:** 9g

Avocado Cilantro Lime Salsa

Prep Time: 15 minutes | **Cook Time:** 0 minutes | **Number of Servings:** 6

Ingredients:

- 3 ripe avocados, diced

- 1 cup cherry tomatoes, halved

- 1/2 cup red onion, finely chopped

- 1/4 cup fresh cilantro, chopped

- 1 jalapeño, seeds removed and finely diced

- Juice of 2 limes

- 1 clove garlic, minced

- Salt and pepper to taste

Instructions:

1. In a large bowl, put together the diced avocados, halved cherry tomatoes, finely chopped red onion, chopped cilantro, and finely diced jalapeño.

2. In a small bowl, whisk together the lime juice and minced garlic.

3. Pour the lime-garlic mixture over the avocado mixture and gently toss to combine.

4. Season the salsa with salt and pepper to taste. Adjust the seasoning as needed.

5. Refrigerate the salsa for at least 30 minutes to allow the flavors to meld.

6. Before serving, give the salsa a gentle stir. Serve chilled with tortilla chips or as a topping for tacos, salads, or grilled vegetables.

Nutritional Information (Per Serving):

- **Carbs:** 10g

- **Fats:** 9g

- **Fiber:** 6g

- **Protein:** 2g

Spiced Edamame Bites

Prep Time: 10 minutes | **Cook Time:** 15 minutes | **Number of Servings:** 4

Ingredients:

- 2 cups frozen edamame, thawed
- 2 tablespoons olive oil
- 1 teaspoon ground cumin
- 1/2 teaspoon smoked paprika
- 1/2 teaspoon garlic powder
- 1/4 teaspoon cayenne pepper
- Salt to taste

Instructions:

1. Preheat the oven to 375°F (190°C).

2. In a bowl, toss the thawed edamame with olive oil, ground cumin, smoked paprika, garlic powder, cayenne pepper, and salt.

3. Spread the seasoned edamame in a single layer on a baking sheet lined with parchment paper.

4. Roast in the preheated oven for 15 minutes or until the edamame are golden and slightly crispy, stirring once halfway through the cooking time.

5. Remove from the oven and let the spiced edamame bites cool for a few minutes before serving.

Nutritional Information (Per Serving):

- **Carbs:** 8g
- **Fats:** 8g
- **Fiber:** 4g
- **Protein:** 10g

Sweet Potato and Turmeric Hummus

Prep Time: 15 minutes | **Cook Time:** 40 minutes | **Number of Servings:** 8

Ingredients:

- 2 medium sweet potatoes, peeled and diced
- 1 can (15 oz) chickpeas, drained and rinsed
- 1/4 cup tahini
- 1/4 cup olive oil
- Juice of 1 lemon

- 2 cloves garlic, minced
- 1 teaspoon ground turmeric
- 1/2 teaspoon ground cumin
- 1/2 teaspoon smoked paprika
- Salt and pepper to taste
- Water (as needed for desired consistency)

Instructions:

1. Preheat the oven to 400°F (200°C).

2. Place the diced sweet potatoes on a baking sheet, drizzle with olive oil, and season with salt and pepper. Roast in the preheated oven for 30-40 minutes or until the sweet potatoes are tender.

3. In a food processor, put together the roasted sweet potatoes, chickpeas, tahini, olive oil, lemon juice, minced garlic, ground turmeric, ground cumin, and smoked paprika.

4. Blend the ingredients until smooth, scraping down the sides as needed. If the hummus is too thick, add water a little at a time until the desired consistency is reached.

5. Season the sweet potato and turmeric hummus with additional salt and pepper to taste.

6. Transfer the hummus to a serving bowl, drizzle with a bit of olive oil, and sprinkle with a pinch of smoked paprika for garnish.

Nutritional Information (Per Serving):

- **Carbs:** 18g
- **Fats:** 8g
- **Fiber:** 4g
- **Protein:** 5g

Kale Chips with Paprika

Prep Time: 10 minutes | **Cook Time:** 15 minutes | **Number of Servings:** 4

Ingredients:

- 1 bunch of kale, stems removed and leaves torn into bite-sized pieces
- 2 tablespoons olive oil
- 1 teaspoon smoked paprika
- 1/2 teaspoon garlic powder
- Salt to taste

Instructions:

1. Preheat the oven to 350°F (175°C).
2. In a large bowl, massage the kale leaves with olive oil until well coated. This helps to tenderize the kale.
3. Sprinkle the torn kale leaves with smoked paprika, garlic powder, and salt. Toss the leaves to ensure an even distribution of the seasonings.
4. Spread the seasoned kale leaves in a single layer on a baking sheet lined with parchment paper.
5. Bake in the preheated oven for 12-15 minutes, or until the kale chips are crisp and the edges are slightly browned. Be sure to check them frequently in the last few minutes to prevent burning.
6. Remove from the oven and let the kale chips cool for a few minutes before serving.

Nutritional Information (Per Serving):

- **Carbs:** 6g
- **Fats:** 5g
- **Fiber:** 2g
- **Protein:** 2g

Roasted Red Pepper and Walnut Dip

Prep Time: 15 minutes | **Cook Time:** 20 minutes | **Number of Servings:** 6

Ingredients:

- 2 large red bell peppers, roasted, peeled, and chopped

- 1 cup walnuts, toasted

- 2 cloves garlic, minced

- 2 tablespoons olive oil

- 1 tablespoon tomato paste

- 1 teaspoon ground cumin

- 1/2 teaspoon smoked paprika

- 1/4 teaspoon cayenne pepper (optional)

- Salt and pepper to taste

- Fresh parsley for garnish

Instructions:

1. Preheat the oven to 425°F (220°C).
2. Place whole red bell peppers on a baking sheet and roast for 15-20 minutes, turning occasionally, until the skin is charred.
3. Transfer the roasted peppers to a bowl, cover with plastic wrap, and let them steam for 10 minutes. Peel off the skin, remove seeds, and chop the flesh.

4. In a food processor, put together the roasted red peppers, toasted walnuts, minced garlic, olive oil, tomato paste, ground cumin, smoked paprika, and cayenne pepper if using.

5. Process the ingredients until the mixture becomes a smooth and creamy dip. If needed, add more olive oil to achieve the desired consistency.

6. Season the dip with salt and pepper to taste.

7. Transfer the roasted red pepper and walnut dip to a serving bowl, garnish with fresh parsley, and refrigerate for at least 30 minutes before serving.

Nutritional Information (Per Serving):

- **Carbs:** 8g

- **Fats:** 17g

- **Fiber:** 3g

- **Protein:** 4g

Sweet Potato and Turmeric Croquettes

Prep Time: 30 minutes | **Cook Time:** 25 minutes | **Number of Servings:** 4

Ingredients:

- 2 large sweet potatoes, peeled and diced

- 1 cup quinoa, cooked

- 1/2 cup breadcrumbs (gluten-free if needed)

- 2 tablespoons ground flaxseeds mixed with 6 tablespoons water (flax eggs)

- 1 teaspoon ground turmeric

- 1 teaspoon smoked paprika

- 1/2 teaspoon ground cumin

- Salt and pepper to taste

- 2 tablespoons olive oil (for cooking)

Instructions:

1. In a small bowl, mix ground flaxseeds with water and let it sit for 5 minutes until it forms a gel-like consistency.
2. Steam the diced sweet potatoes until they are fork-tender. Mash them in a large bowl.
3. To the mashed sweet potatoes, add cooked quinoa, breadcrumbs, flax eggs, ground turmeric, smoked paprika, ground cumin, salt, and pepper. Mix adequately until all ingredients are evenly combined.
4. Shape the mixture into croquettes. If the mixture is too sticky, wet your hands with water to make shaping easier.
5. Heat olive oil in a skillet over medium heat.
6. Place the croquettes in the skillet and cook for 4-5 minutes on each side or until they are golden brown and crispy.
7. Once cooked, transfer the sweet potato and turmeric croquettes to a plate lined with paper towels to absorb any excess oil.
8. Serve the croquettes warm, and enjoy!

Nutritional Information (Per Serving):

- **Carbs:** 45g

- **Fats:** 10g

- **Fiber:** 7g

- **Protein:** 8g

<u>Turmeric Spiced Pumpkin Seeds</u>

Prep Time: 10 minutes | **Cook Time:** 15 minutes | **Number of Servings:** 6

Ingredients:

- 2 cups raw pumpkin seeds
- 1 tablespoon olive oil
- 1 teaspoon ground turmeric
- 1/2 teaspoon ground cumin
- 1/2 teaspoon smoked paprika
- 1/4 teaspoon cayenne pepper (optional)
- Salt to taste

Instructions:

1. Preheat the oven to 325°F (163°C).
2. In a bowl, toss the raw pumpkin seeds with olive oil until well coated.
3. In a small bowl, mix ground turmeric, ground cumin, smoked paprika, and cayenne pepper if using.
4. Sprinkle the spice mixture over the pumpkin seeds and toss until the seeds are evenly coated with the spices.
5. Spread the seasoned pumpkin seeds in a single layer on a baking sheet lined with parchment paper.
6. Roast in the preheated oven for 15 minutes, stirring halfway through the cooking time, until the pumpkin seeds are golden brown.
7. Remove from the oven and sprinkle with salt to taste. Allow the seeds to cool before serving.

Nutritional Information (Per Serving):

- **Carbs:** 4g
- **Fats:** 14g
- **Fiber:** 2g
- **Protein:** 10g

Cauliflower Buffalo Bites with Cashew Ranch

Prep Time: 20 minutes | **Cook Time:** 25 minutes | **Number of Servings:** 4

Ingredients:

For Cauliflower Buffalo Bites:

- 1 large head cauliflower, cut into florets
- 1 cup chickpea flour
- 1 cup water
- 1 teaspoon garlic powder
- 1 teaspoon onion powder
- 1/2 teaspoon smoked paprika
- 1/2 teaspoon cumin
- Salt and pepper to taste
- 1 cup buffalo sauce
- 2 tablespoons olive oil (for baking)

For Cashew Ranch:

- 1 cup raw cashews, soaked in water for 2 hours
- 1/2 cup water
- 2 tablespoons lemon juice
- 1 clove garlic
- 1 tablespoon fresh dill, chopped
- 1 tablespoon fresh chives, chopped
- Salt and pepper to taste

Instructions:

1. Preheat the oven to 450°F (232°C).
2. In a large bowl, whisk together chickpea flour, water, garlic powder, onion powder, smoked paprika, cumin, salt, and pepper to create a batter.
3. Dip each cauliflower floret into the batter, ensuring it's fully coated, and place it on a baking sheet lined with parchment paper.
4. Drizzle olive oil over the battered cauliflower.
5. Bake in the preheated oven for 20-25 minutes or until golden brown, flipping halfway through.
6. In a separate bowl, toss the baked cauliflower in buffalo sauce until well coated.
7. In a blender, combine soaked cashews, water, lemon juice, garlic, dill, chives, salt, and pepper. Blend until smooth and creamy.
8. Serve the cauliflower buffalo bites with cashew ranch on the side for dipping.

Nutritional Information (Per Serving):

- **Carbs:** 32g
- **Fats:** 18g
- **Fiber:** 6g
- **Protein:** 12g

Edamame and Mint Guacamole

Prep Time: 15 minutes | **Cook Time:** 0 minutes | **Number of Servings:** 6

Ingredients:

- 3 ripe avocados, peeled and mashed

- 1 cup edamame, shelled and cooked

- 1/2 cup red onion, finely chopped

- 1/4 cup fresh mint leaves, finely chopped

- 2 cloves garlic, minced

- Juice of 2 limes

- Salt and pepper to taste

- Cherry tomatoes for garnish (optional)

Instructions:

1. In a large bowl, put together the mashed avocados with shelled and cooked edamame.

2. Add finely chopped red onion, finely chopped fresh mint leaves, and minced garlic to the bowl.

3. Squeeze the juice of two limes into the mixture.

4. Season the guacamole with salt and pepper to taste. Mix adequately to combine all ingredients.

5. Garnish the guacamole with cherry tomatoes if desired.

6. Serve the edamame and mint guacamole immediately with tortilla chips or as a topping for tacos, salads, or grilled vegetables.

Nutritional Information (Per Serving):

- **Carbs:** 12g

- **Fats:** 15g

- **Fiber:** 7g

- **Protein:** 5g

Sun-Dried Tomato and Basil Hummus

Prep Time: 15 minutes | **Cook Time:** 0 minutes | **Number of Servings:** 8

Ingredients:

- 1 can (15 oz) chickpeas, drained and rinsed
- 1/2 cup sun-dried tomatoes (not in oil), soaked in warm water
- 1/4 cup fresh basil leaves
- 1/4 cup tahini
- 1/4 cup olive oil
- Juice of 1 lemon
- 2 cloves garlic, minced
- 1/2 teaspoon ground cumin
- Salt and pepper to taste
- Water (as needed for desired consistency)

Instructions:

1. Soak sun-dried tomatoes in warm water for about 10 minutes to soften them. Drain and set aside.
2. In a food processor, combine drained and rinsed chickpeas, soaked sun-dried tomatoes, fresh basil leaves, tahini, olive oil, lemon juice, minced garlic, and ground cumin.
3. Blend the ingredients until smooth, scraping down the sides as needed. If the hummus is too thick, add water a little at a time until the desired consistency is reached.
4. Season the sun-dried tomato and basil hummus with salt and pepper to taste.
5. Transfer the hummus to a serving bowl and drizzle with a bit of olive oil for garnish.
6. Garnish with additional fresh basil leaves if desired.

Nutritional Information (Per Serving):

- **Carbs:** 14g
- **Fats:** 10g
- **Fiber:** 4g
- **Protein:** 5g

Crispy Turmeric Baked Kale Chips

Prep Time: 10 minutes | **Cook Time:** 15 minutes | **Number of Servings:** 4

Ingredients:

- 1 bunch of kale, stems removed and torn into bite-sized pieces
- 2 tablespoons olive oil
- 1 teaspoon ground turmeric
- 1/2 teaspoon garlic powder
- 1/2 teaspoon onion powder
- 1/4 teaspoon cayenne pepper (optional)
- Salt to taste

Instructions:

1. Preheat the oven to 350°F (175°C).
2. Wash the kale leaves thoroughly and ensure they are completely dry.
3. Take out the stems and tear the leaves into bite-sized pieces.
4. In a large bowl, massage the kale pieces with olive oil until well coated.
5. Sprinkle ground turmeric, garlic powder, onion powder, and cayenne pepper if using. Toss to ensure even coating.
6. Spread the seasoned kale in a single layer on a baking sheet lined with parchment paper.
7. Bake in the preheated oven for 12-15 minutes or until the kale chips are crisp and the edges are slightly browned. Check frequently in the last few minutes to prevent burning.
8. Remove from the oven and sprinkle with salt to taste. Allow the chips to cool for a few minutes before serving.

Nutritional Information (Per Serving):

- **Carbs:** 8g
- **Fats:** 5g
- **Fiber:** 2g
- **Protein:** 3g

Turmeric Hemp Seed Energy Bites

Prep Time: 15 minutes | **Cook Time:** 0 minutes | **Number of Servings:** 12

Ingredients:

- 1 cup rolled oats
- 1/2 cup almond butter
- 1/3 cup maple syrup
- 1/4 cup hemp seeds
- 1/4 cup ground flaxseeds
- 1 teaspoon ground turmeric
- 1/2 teaspoon cinnamon
- 1/2 teaspoon vanilla extract
- A pinch of sea salt

Instructions:

1. In a large bowl, combine rolled oats, almond butter, maple syrup, hemp seeds, ground flaxseeds, ground turmeric, cinnamon, vanilla extract, and a pinch of sea salt.
2. Mix the ingredients thoroughly until well combined.
3. Place the mixture in the refrigerator for about 30 minutes to firm up.
4. Once chilled, take small portions of the mixture and roll them into bite-sized balls.
5. Store the turmeric hemp seed energy bites in an airtight container in the refrigerator.
6. Serve chilled and enjoy as a nutritious snack.

Nutritional Information (Per Serving - 1 Energy Bite):

- **Carbs:** 13g
- **Fats:** 7g
- **Fiber:** 2g
- **Protein:** 4g

Crispy Baked Turmeric Artichoke Hearts

Prep Time: 15 minutes | **Cook Time:** 25 minutes | **Number of Servings:** 4

Ingredients:

- 2 cans (14 oz each) artichoke hearts, drained and halved
- 1/2 cup breadcrumbs (gluten-free if needed)
- 1/4 cup nutritional yeast
- 1 teaspoon ground turmeric
- 1/2 teaspoon garlic powder
- 1/2 teaspoon onion powder
- Salt and pepper to taste
- 2 tablespoons olive oil

Instructions:

1. Preheat the oven to 400°F (200°C).
2. Drain the artichoke hearts and cut them in half.
3. In a bowl, combine breadcrumbs, nutritional yeast, ground turmeric, garlic powder, onion powder, salt, and pepper.
4. Toss the halved artichoke hearts in the coating mixture until they are evenly coated.
5. Place the coated artichoke hearts on a baking sheet lined with parchment paper.
6. Drizzle olive oil over the artichoke hearts to help them crisp up in the oven.
7. Bake in the preheated oven for 25 minutes or until the artichoke hearts are golden and crispy.
8. Serve the crispy baked turmeric artichoke hearts warm as a delicious appetizer or snack.

Nutritional Information (Per Serving):

- **Carbs:** 15g
- **Fats:** 8g
- **Fiber:** 5g
- **Protein:** 4g

Miso Glazed Edamame Pods

Prep Time: 10 minutes | **Cook Time:** 10 minutes | **Number of Servings:** 4

Ingredients:

- 2 cups edamame pods
- 2 tablespoons white miso paste
- 1 tablespoon maple syrup
- 1 tablespoon rice vinegar
- 1 teaspoon sesame oil
- 1 teaspoon grated ginger
- 1 clove garlic, minced
- 1 tablespoon sesame seeds (for garnish)
- Chopped green onions (for garnish)

Instructions:

1. Boil edamame pods in salted water for about 5-7 minutes or until tender. Drain and set aside.
2. In a small bowl, whisk together white miso paste, maple syrup, rice vinegar, sesame oil, grated ginger, and minced garlic.
3. In a pan over medium heat, add the boiled edamame pods and pour the miso glaze over them. Stir adequately to ensure even coating.
4. Cook for an additional 3-5 minutes, allowing the miso glaze to caramelize slightly and coat the edamame pods.
5. Sprinkle sesame seeds and chopped green onions over the glazed edamame pods for added flavor and visual appeal.
6. Transfer the miso glazed edamame pods to a serving dish and serve warm.

Nutritional Information (Per Serving):

- **Carbs:** 14g
- **Fats:** 5g
- **Fiber:** 5g
- **Protein:** 9g

Spicy Turmeric Popcorn

Prep Time: 5 minutes | **Cook Time:** 5 minutes | **Number of Servings:** 4

Ingredients:

- 1/2 cup popcorn kernels
- 3 tablespoons coconut oil
- 1 teaspoon ground turmeric
- 1/2 teaspoon smoked paprika
- 1/4 teaspoon cayenne pepper
- Salt to taste
- Optional: nutritional yeast for added flavor

Instructions:

1. Pop the popcorn kernels using your preferred method (air popper, stovetop, or microwave).
2. In a small pan, melt coconut oil over low heat. Add ground turmeric, smoked paprika, and cayenne pepper to the melted coconut oil. Stir adequately to create a spice mixture.
3. Drizzle the spiced coconut oil mixture over the popped popcorn. Ensure the popcorn is well coated by gently tossing it.
4. Sprinkle salt over the spiced popcorn to taste. Add nutritional yeast if desired for an extra layer of flavor.
5. Toss the popcorn again to evenly distribute the spices. Serve immediately.

Nutritional Information (Per Serving):

- **Carbs:** 18g
- **Fats:** 14g
- **Fiber:** 4g
- **Protein:** 2g

Almond and Turmeric Stuffed Grape Leaves

Prep Time: 30 minutes | **Cook Time:** 30 minutes | **Number of Servings:** 6

Ingredients:

- 1 jar grape leaves in brine, drained and rinsed
- 1 cup short-grain brown rice, cooked
- 1/2 cup almonds, finely chopped
- 1/4 cup fresh parsley, finely chopped
- 1/4 cup fresh dill, finely chopped
- 1 small red onion, finely chopped
- 2 cloves garlic, minced
- 1 teaspoon ground turmeric
- 1/2 teaspoon ground cumin
- 1/4 cup olive oil
- Juice of 2 lemons
- Salt and pepper to taste
- Lemon wedges for serving

Instructions:

1. Carefully remove grape leaves from the jar, unfold, and rinse under cold water. Trim any tough stems.
2. In a large bowl, combine cooked short-grain brown rice, finely chopped almonds, finely chopped fresh parsley, finely chopped fresh dill, finely chopped red onion, minced garlic, ground turmeric, and ground cumin.
3. Add olive oil, lemon juice, salt, and pepper to the filling mixture. Mix adequately to combine all ingredients.
4. Place a grape leaf on a flat surface, shiny side down. Spoon a small amount of the filling onto the center of the leaf. Fold the sides of the leaf over the filling and roll it tightly from the bottom to the top.
5. Place the stuffed grape leaves in a wide pot, seam side down, packing them tightly.
6. Add enough water to the pot to cover the grape leaves. Place a heavy plate or lid on top to keep the grape leaves from unraveling during cooking. Simmer over low heat for about 30 minutes or until the grape leaves are tender.
7. Allow the stuffed grape leaves to cool slightly before serving. Serve with lemon wedges.

Nutritional Information (Per Serving):

- **Carbs:** 30g
- **Fats:** 12g
- **Fiber:** 5g
- **Protein:** 6g

Mediterranean Roasted Red Pepper and Walnut Dip

Prep Time: 15 minutes | **Cook Time:** 20 minutes | **Number of Servings:** 8

Ingredients:

- 2 large red bell peppers
- 1 cup walnuts, toasted
- 1/4 cup olive oil
- 2 cloves garlic, minced
- 1 teaspoon ground cumin
- 1 teaspoon smoked paprika
- 1/2 teaspoon cayenne pepper (optional)
- Salt and pepper to taste
- Juice of 1 lemon
- 1/4 cup fresh parsley, chopped (for garnish)

Instructions:

1. Preheat the oven broiler. Place red bell peppers on a baking sheet and broil, turning occasionally, until the skins are charred and blistered. Remove from the oven, place in a bowl, cover with plastic wrap, and let them steam for 10 minutes. Peel, seed, and dice the roasted red peppers.
2. In a dry pan over medium heat, toast the walnuts until fragrant. Be careful not to burn them. Let them cool.
3. In a food processor, put together the roasted red peppers, toasted walnuts, olive oil, minced garlic, ground cumin, smoked paprika, cayenne pepper if using, salt, and pepper.
4. Blend the ingredients until smooth, scraping down the sides as needed.
5. Add the juice of one lemon to the dip and blend again until well combined.
6. Taste and adjust salt, pepper, and lemon juice as needed.
7. Transfer the dip to a serving bowl, garnish with chopped fresh parsley, and serve.

Nutritional Information (Per Serving):

- **Carbs:** 7g
- **Fats:** 18g
- **Fiber:** 2g
- **Protein:** 4g

Chapter 9: Tips for a Sustainable Anti-Inflammatory Vegan Lifestyle

Meal Planning and Preparation

Adopting a sustainable, anti-inflammatory vegan lifestyle requires thoughtful planning and preparation. Here are some strategies to help you stay organized and make the most of your meals:

1. **Plan Your Meals:** Allocate a specific period each week to plan your meals. This guarantees you all the necessary ingredients and keeps you on course. To keep your meals exciting and nutritionally balanced, consider incorporating various colors and textures of ingredients.

2. **Batch Cooking:** At the start of the week, prepare large batches of staple foods, like grains, legumes, and roasted vegetables. Store them in airtight containers in the fridge for easy access when assembling meals.

3. **Prepare Ingredients in Advance:** Chop vegetables, wash greens, and portion out snacks beforehand. This makes it easy to whip up quick, healthy meals and reduces prep time during the workweek.

4. **Use Flexible Recipes:** Choose recipes that can be easily adapted based on what you have on hand. Versatile recipes, such as salads, grain bowls, and stir-fries, can accommodate various ingredients, cutting down on waste and adding excitement to your meals.

5. **Invest in High-Quality Storage:** To store prepped ingredients and leftovers, use silicone bags, glass jars, and reusable containers. This lessens your dependency on single-use plastics and keeps your food fresh.

6. **Make a Weekly Menu:** Post your menu for the week in your kitchen. This visual reminder encourages you to stick to your meal plan and can motivate you to experiment with different recipes and ingredients.

Stocking Your Pantry

A well-stocked pantry is the cornerstone of a sustainable, anti-inflammatory vegan diet. The following tips can help you keep a pantry that supports your health objectives:

1. **Essential Grains:** Stock up on a range of whole grains, including barley, quinoa, brown rice, and oats. These nutritious, versatile grains can serve as a base for various recipes.

2. **Legumes and Beans:** Keep a supply of dried or canned beans and lentils on hand. They are excellent plant-based protein and fiber sources and can be used in soups, stews, salads, and more.

3. **Nuts and Seeds:** You can add healthy fats, proteins, and texture to your meals by eating nuts and seeds like almonds, walnuts, chia seeds, flaxseeds, and hemp seeds. To keep them fresh, store them in airtight containers.

4. **Healthy Oils:** Olive, coconut, and avocado oils are essential for cooking and dressing salads. They're rich in beneficial fats which support an anti-inflammatory diet.

5. **Herbs and Spices:** You can enhance the flavor and anti-inflammatory qualities of your food by incorporating a variety of herbs and spices, like cumin, turmeric, ginger, garlic, and cinnamon.

6. **Nutritional Yeast:** A staple of vegan cooking, this versatile ingredient gives food a cheesy flavor and is a fantastic source of B vitamins.

7. **Canned Goods:** Stock your pantry with canned tomatoes, coconut milk, and vegetable broth. These are handy for making quick and flavorful sauces, stews, and soups.

8. **Frozen Fruits and Vegetables:** Keeping a variety of frozen produce on hand guarantees you always have wholesome ingredients on hand, even when fresh options are scarce.

Dining Out and Social Occurrences

Navigating social situations and dining out can be challenging for someone following an anti-inflammatory vegan diet. Here are some tips to keep you on course:

1. **Research Restaurants:** Before heading out, look up menus online for vegan and anti-inflammatory options at restaurants. Many restaurants serve plant-based meals or are open to special requests.

2. **Communicate Your Needs:** Please do not hesitate to let the chef or waiter know about your dietary preferences. Most restaurants are willing to modify their food offerings to meet your requirements.

3. **Be Prepared:** When attending social events or gatherings, propose to bring a dish that satisfies your dietary needs. This guarantees you will have your ideal food on hand and potentially introduce others to the vegan-centric, anti-inflammatory lifestyle as well.

4. **Snack Wisely:** When you're out and about, keep anti-inflammatory snacks like fruit, nuts, and seeds on hand. This will prevent you from acting on impulse and choosing fewer options when you're hungry.

5. **Remain Hydrated:** Drinking water at various times during the day makes you feel full and reduces cravings. When dining out, drink water or herbal teas instead of sugary or alcoholic beverages.

Maintaining Consistency and Motivation

It takes dedication and drive to keep up a sustainable anti-inflammatory vegan lifestyle. The following strategies can help you in staying on course:

1. **Set Realistic Goals:** Begin with feasible goals and progressively expand upon them. Small steps can result in enduring changes, whether trying one new recipe a week or increasing the number of whole foods in your diet.

2. **Monitor Your Progress:** Use an app or a journal to track your meals, energy levels, and general state of health daily. Monitoring your progress can serve as a strong motivator.

3. **Find Support:** Connect with people who have similar nutritional objectives, join neighborhood or online communities, or both. Support networks can offer accountability and encouragement.

4. **Educate Yourself:** Continuously learn about the benefits of an anti-inflammatory vegan diet. You'll be more driven to persevere if you understand the positive impact it has on your health.

5. **Celebrate Your Successes:** Whether it's perfecting a new dish or finishing a week's worth of meal prep, reward yourself when you hit milestones. Rewarding yourself for your accomplishments reinforces positive conduct.

6. **Stay Flexible:** Since life can be unpredictable, staying flexible is critical. Don't be too hard on yourself if you make mistakes or encounter difficulties. Focus on recovering and growing from the event.

7. **Prioritize Self-Care:** Make time for mental and physical wellness practices like exercise, meditation, and quality sleep. A holistic approach to health can strengthen your dedication to an anti-inflammatory vegan lifestyle.

By implementing these tips, you can create a sustainable, anti-inflammatory vegan lifestyle that promotes your general wellness and health. Remember that the journey is as important as the destination, and every positive change you make leads to a healthier and happier future.

Chapter 10: Frequently Asked Questions

Common Concerns Addressed

Q: Will an anti-inflammatory vegan diet provide me with enough protein?

A: Plant-based foods, including beans, lentils, tofu, tempeh, nuts, and seeds, are excellent protein sources. You can easily achieve your protein needs by including a variety of these foods in your diet.

Q: Is getting sufficient vitamins and minerals challenging when following a vegan diet?

A: Not at all. You can obtain all the vitamins and minerals your body needs with a carefully designed vegan diet. Good sources of essential vitamins and minerals include leafy greens, legumes, nuts, seeds, and fortified meals.

Q: Will I lose weight on an anti-inflammatory vegan diet?

A: An anti-inflammatory vegan diet can help you lose weight, particularly if you emphasize whole, nutrient-rich foods and minimize processed foods. Individual outcomes, however, can differ based on factors like activity level and calorie consumption.

Q: Can an anti-inflammatory vegan diet help correct digestive problems?

A: Yes, many people find that adopting an anti-inflammatory vegan diet can improve digestive health. Plant-based diets' high fiber content can improve gut health and aid digestion.

Tips for Transitioning

Do it Gradually: Transitioning to a vegan diet that reduces inflammation doesn't have to be abrupt. Begin by adding more plant-based meals to your routine and gradually decreasing your consumption of animal products.

Educate Yourself: Learn about the benefits of an anti-inflammatory vegan diet and become acquainted with various plant-based protein sources, cooking methods, and ingredient substitutions.

Try out different recipes: Explore new recipes and flavors to add excitement and satisfaction to your meals. There is a wealth of vegan recipes available online and in cookbooks to ignite your culinary adventure.

Seek Support: Connecting with online communities or local vegan groups can offer valuable support and advice as you make the switch to a plant-based diet.

Maintaining Balance and Variety

Embrace a Diverse Array of Colors: Incorporate a wide selection of vibrant fruits and vegetables into your diet to ensure a rich assortment of nutrients and antioxidants.

Diversify Your Protein Sources: Vary your plant-based protein sources by including beans, lentils, tofu, tempeh, and seitan in your diet. This will help you obtain a well-rounded amino acid profile.

Incorporate Whole Grains: Include a variety of whole grains, such as quinoa, brown rice, oats, and barley, in your meals to ensure you receive a good amount of fiber, vitamins, and minerals.

Don't Forget Healthy Fats: Remember to incorporate sources of healthy fats, such as avocados, nuts, seeds, and olive oil, into your diet. These can help support brain health and reduce inflammation.

Stay Hydrated: Drink plenty of water throughout the day to stay hydrated. This will help support digestion, nutrient absorption, and overall health.

Pay attention to your body: Be alert and mindful of the effects of various foods on your body and adjust your diet based on those observations. Every individual has a distinct body, so it is crucial to discover what suits you the most.

We've designed this FAQ section to help you achieve a sustainable, anti-inflammatory vegan lifestyle by addressing common concerns, providing transitional tips, and offering strategies for maintaining balance and variety. Keep in mind that the focus should be on progress rather than perfection. Take the time to appreciate the journey of discovering new foods and flavors, and be gentle with yourself along the way.

Conclusion

Congratulations on completing ***"The Complete Anti-Inflammatory Vegan Cookbook"*** by Amanda K. Sanders! This cookbook gives you the necessary knowledge and tools to adopt a sustainable, plant-based diet that promotes health and vitality. By incorporating foods with anti-inflammatory properties into your meals and making thoughtful choices, you've taken a proactive step towards a healthier, inflammation-free future.

Consistency is crucial as you embark on your anti-inflammatory vegan journey. Acknowledge and celebrate your achievements, whether they're minor changes to your diet or significant strides in improving your health. Stay connected with the vegan and anti-inflammatory communities for support and inspiration, and continue to explore new recipes and ingredients to keep your meals exciting and nourishing.

Above all, pay attention to your body and respect its needs. Everyone has their unique qualities, so it's crucial to discover what methods are most effective for you. Whether you're interested in managing inflammation, enhancing your immune system, or enjoying flavorful, plant-based meals, this cookbook offers the knowledge to make well-informed decisions and nurture your body from within.

We appreciate you joining us on this adventure. May your meals be flavorful, your health thriving, and your compassion limitless. Here's to a lifetime of enjoying delicious, anti-inflammatory vegan meals!

Recipes Index

Lemon Rosemary White Bean Soup 24

Lemon Thyme Roasted Sweet Potatoes 78

Lemon Turmeric Roasted Fingerling Potatoes 84

Lentil and Vegetable Stir-Fry 51

Lentil Walnut Burger with Avocado Aioli 60

M

Mango Avocado Black Bean Salad 47

Mango Basil Summer Salad 36

Mango Ginger Green Tea Infusion 90

Mango Turmeric Chia Seed Pudding Smoothie 98

Mediterranean Lentil and Artichoke Salad 40

Mediterranean Roasted Red Pepper and Walnut Dip 124

Miso Glazed Edamame Pods 121

Miso Glazed Eggplant Slices 75

Moroccan Spiced Eggplant and Couscous Skillet 61

Moroccan Spiced Lentil and Eggplant Casserole 64

O

Orange Fennel Detox Salad 42

Orange Turmeric Mango Smoothie Bowl 105

P

Papaya Turmeric Immunity Elixir 102

Pineapple Basil Anti-Inflammatory Cooler 104

Pineapple Mint Coconut Water Refresher 97

Pineapple Turmeric Smoothie 88

Portobello Mushroom and Spinach Stuffed Peppers 57

Q

Quinoa and Avocado Anti-Inflammatory Salad 31

Quinoa and Black Bean Stuffed Bell Peppers 67

Quinoa Minestrone with Kale and Cannellini Beans 29

Quinoa Vegetable Turmeric Congee 21

Quinoa-Stuffed Portobello Mushrooms 53

R

Raspberry Turmeric Ginger Smoothie 100

Red Lentil and Kale Anti-Inflammatory Stew 18

Roasted Beet and Walnut Arugula Salad 33

Roasted Brussels Sprouts and Pomegranate Salad 37

Roasted Cauliflower and Cumin Chickpea Salad 44

Roasted Garlic and Herb Quinoa 77

Roasted Red Pepper and Walnut Dip 112

S

Sesame Crusted Tofu with Turmeric Citrus Glaze 56

Smoky Turmeric Grilled Portobello Mushrooms 65

Spaghetti Squash with Roasted Tomato Sauce 52

Spaghetti Squash with Spinach and Pine Nut Pesto 66

Spiced Chickpea and Zucchini Fritters 86

Spiced Edamame Bites 109

Spiced Pumpkin and Lentil Stew 25

Spicy Black Bean and Spinach Detox Soup 22

Spicy Turmeric Popcorn 122

Spinach and White Bean Detox Soup 14

Spinach Strawberry Walnut Salad with Balsamic Vinaigrette 48

Spirulina Citrus Superfood Smoothie 99

Sun-Dried Tomato and Basil Hummus 117

Sweet Potato and Turmeric Croquettes 113

Sweet Potato and Turmeric Hummus 110

Sweet Potato Ginger Stew 13

T

Thai-Inspired Lemongrass Coconut Soup 27

Turmeric Cauliflower Mash 70

W

Z

www.ingramcontent.com/pod-product-compliance
Lightning Source LLC
Chambersburg PA
CBHW081214260726
48653CB00010BA/3652